WOMEN OF COLOR IN A WORLD APART

Care, whether viewed as acts of civility, acts of compassion and skill, or acts of close personal interaction, is the fundamental process by which society perpetuates and recreates itself. Despite social need and the undeniable benefit of occupations such as Certified Nursing Assistants (CNAs), these workers—mostly female and disproportionally from minority groups—face very low wages, a notable lack of respect, and little public recognition of their abilities. The United States is experiencing what experts call a crisis of care with a current and growing shortage of nurses and CNAs. In U.S. Nursing Centers, the demand for Certified Nursing Assistants, the largest group of employees who operate on the front line of health care, is expected to grow exponentially due to dramatic increases in population aging.

Over the course of a year and a half, Anne K. Vittoria examined the meaning and social construction of care work on an Alzheimer's Pavilion located in a geriatric facility in the mid-western United States. Through in-depth ethnographic research focused on the local culture and logic of care, Vittoria documents that, when given autonomy in their daily work in an institution, CNAs and the LPN Charge Nurse constructed a systematic body of knowledge and created a language of care—forging a "different" model of personal care in resistance to the medical model of care. This book challenges the assumptions of the outside world that low-level workers are alienated from their work and have minimal skills. Paradoxically, the Pavilion is both a refuge and a site of struggle for the CNAs; they desire to create a world that is the antithesis of the world in which they live on the outside. *Women of Color in a World Apart* provides a public forum for the voices of women of color, the development of concepts, and a practical as well as theoretical language of care that could be transformational in connecting the meanings of care with the organization of care.

Anne K. Vittoria is Associate Professor of Sociology, Gender Studies, Social Psychology, Aging, and Consumer Society at the State University of New York Cortland. Support for this research and writing came from the National Alzheimer's Association and the SUNY Dresher Award.

WOMEN OF COLOR IN A WORLD APART

An Ethnography of Care Workers and Dementia

Anne K. Vittoria

Routledge
Taylor & Francis Group
NEW YORK AND LONDON

First published 2021
by Routledge
52 Vanderbilt Avenue, New York, NY 10017

and by Routledge
2 Park Square, Milton Park, Abingdon, Oxon OX14 4RN

Routledge is an imprint of the Taylor & Francis Group, an informa business

Library of Congress Cataloging-in-Publication Data
A catalog record for this title has been requested

ISBN: 978-0-367-37080-0 (hbk)
ISBN: 978-0-367-37081-7 (pbk)
ISBN: 978-0-429-35259-1 (ebk)

Typeset in Bembo
by Newgen Publishing UK

To my parents Mary and Benjamin
And to my grandfather, Jacob Thompson Perkins, the consummate newspaper man, who first inspired me to write.
And to my husband, Theodore John Vittoria, who inspired me, unfailingly, to grow as a person.

CONTENTS

ACKNOWLEDGMENTS

I want to extend a bountiful thank you to the Certified Nursing Assistants, the Charge Nurse and the residents of the Alzheimer's Pavilion for accepting me as part of their world for a year and a half. They did not know what to expect and neither did I. The coming of trust was the conduit to understanding. I am indebted to the residents who are deceased now for their uniqueness and spritely comments amid confusion and searching. I am grateful to the CNAs and Charge Nurse for their willingness to talk candidly about their work and allow me to bear witness to their actions. On a several occasions, they volunteered to meet after hours and reflect on the day's happenings over a big pot of coffee. As well, I extend sincere appreciation to the members of the residents' families who gave their time for extended interviews about their experiences with their loved one and impressions of the care work of the CNAs.

Mentors have given many kinds of strategic support during the process of writing this book. As I wrestled with frustrations and blocks, they listened, gave of their time and insights as scholars and sojourners in my life. First and foremost, colleague, mentor and valued friend, Mary Zimmerman, has read the full manuscript several times offering excellent critiques for making the editing and structure of the book clear. A creative sociologist, she has been steadfast in her belief in my work and extraordinary in sharing her time and thoughts, all of which have made this a stronger book. Throughout, her intuitive grasp of the substance of my book has been a great asset.

I thank the early mentors (later friends) who influenced me significantly and opened new worlds: the late Harold Orbach who made social theory come alive; Robert Atchley, who urged me to value my own experience and use my creativity; Carol A.B. Warren, who first introduced me to qualitative methods as a way of studying the human community; Robert Antonio, who exuded a passion for sociological theory; and David Seamon, who gave me a "language of place." Over the years, Michael Flaherty, from afar, provided crucial insights related to my developing the manuscript, and that most essential of gifts, encouragement for a sometimes flagging spirit. I am grateful for steadfast friends and colleagues who have accompanied me on this journey and offered support—each in his or her own way—Eugenia Lasley, Penelope Valmassoi, Lisi Krall, Tiantian Zheng, Kassim Kone, Raymond Collings, Leslie Eaton, Jamie Dangler, Kathryn Kramer, Toni Calasanti, Pamela Mayberry, Warren and Betty Jane Robinson, Lyn Norris-Baker, John Demand, Edith Stunkel, Stephani Robson, Paul Windley, Howard Stevenson and Bonnie Johnson. Robin Hizey, who died too young, was a tremendous help to me in transcribing many transcripts. I could not have done it without her. She was a loyal friend and lovely human being whom we all miss.

A very special thank you goes to those colleagues who read the manuscript at different stages and gave wise counsel and detailed suggestions for improving the substance and direction of the narrative. I am indebted to Joel Savishinsky for his meticulous reading and insightful three-page comments in the late stages of my writing. I thank my colleagues, Tiantian Zheng and Kassim Kone who read a very early draft.

I would like to thank an anonymous reviewer who shall be the champion of "less is more." I am grateful for his belief in this project, his patience when I sorely needed it, and his stewardship along the way. Through the process of working with this reviewer, I came to a true understanding of ethnographic writing because of how well he knew it.

Jen Hinchliffe, my copyeditor, has been outstanding. She has an incomparable eye for detail and knows her publisher's style at all times. Furthermore, she involves herself in the rhythm of the book's narrative; she reads in-depth which allows her to catch mistakes, understand and honor nuances in the author's thought, and choice of words. She strives for excellence on every page and is an indefatigable professional.

I also want to thank Dean Birkenkamp, Senior Editor of Sociology at Routledge for his strong belief in the manuscript, his consistent thoughtfulness and geniality in our association, his suggestions for the book, his patience, and his "listening ear."

Finally, I want to extend a deep appreciation to the triumvirate without whose insights this book would not have come to fruition, H. Lerner, W. Carney, and P. Karr-S. who were part of the quest to understand what appeared to be ineffable.

Portions of Chapter 3 were originally published in "Preserving Selves: Identity Work and Dementia," *Research on Aging*, 20 (1) and reprinted with permission. Portions of Chapter 8 were originally published in "Our Own Little Language: Naming and the Social Construction of Alzheimer's Disease," *Symbolic Interaction*, 22 (4).

INTRODUCTION

In a business-like manner, a substitute Certified Medication Technician, (CMT) is rolling a cart down the nursing home corridor dispensing medicine. Resident Marge Jacobs[1] is moving swiftly toward the cart when the CMT eyes her and shrieks, "Don't you spit on me, stop that spittin'." The two Certified Nurse Assistants[2] (CNAs) I am talking with, Justine and Arnella, spin around at the same moment that CNA Glenda approaches from the right. Standing her ground in front of the medicine cart, Marge does her characteristic "jig." She moves her legs up and down to her own special rhythm, hands clutching her skirt almost as though she were ready to dance if a willing partner appeared. Without missing a beat, Glenda cups her hand under Marge's elbow, pirouettes 180 degrees so that their backs are to the substitute aide, and adroitly dance-steps the two of them away. All the while, Glenda whispers softly, "Come on, Marge, let's go over here ..."

Instantly, Justine jumps up and walks toward the substitute aide. "Just what happened here?" she asks in a heated tone. The substitute aide answers, "she spit on me." "Well I don't know if she did or not but we don't talk to our residents the way you just did. No sir-ee. We, ah, do things just a LIT…tle differently down here."

With a look of chagrin mixed with anger, the aide turns on her heels and quickly heads down the corridor, stops only to enter the code to release the locked doors, and disappears. Justine shakes her head and says to no one in particular, "It just makes me so mad and gives me a headache. When you come on our floor, you got to respect us, you got to respect our residents. Things work differently down here."

"Here" is the first-floor garden level in the Helen Wise Alzheimer's Dementia[3] Pavilion at Starrmount Geriatric Center.[4] CNA Justine King conveys with her tone of voice, and an upward turn of her head, just how large this "little" difference might be. In her briefing of a temporary CNA from another floor, Justine is no-holds-barred explicit in her expectations. She is speaking also to an audience beyond the world of the Pavilion, to society in general. This audience must realize that possessing the numerical code to open the large doors marking the transition from the outside world into the world of the Alzheimer's Pavilion does not immediately unlock its social world and therapeutic milieu. That requires something more, which lies beyond the technical expertise that all CNAs lay some claim to as paraprofessionals.[5] This care environment is "a world apart" in multiple ways. The following chapters explore these features and social dynamics, at the same time suggesting why the unit has evolved this way. My analysis also contains important implications for how societies might more humanely structure dementia care work as well as long-term care work in general.

The episode at Starrmount gave me a tiny window into the construction of a world of care, a complex world I would come to know over my eighteen months of ethnographic fieldwork[6] at this urban geriatric facility in the mid-western United States. Justine's emphatic words, "No sir-ee. We, ah, do things just a LIT… tle differently down here" intrigued me. I set out to find out what she meant.

Care work[7] in the United States and other affluent nations is highly valued by the individuals who receive it, and the work receives generic cultural support. Jobs such as nursing assistant, home health aide and child daycare worker are vital to the quality of life for millions of older persons and young children, making possible successful social and economic arrangements within many American families. Despite social need and the undeniable contribution of these occupations, workers in such positions face low pay and a notable lack of social status.[8] For these paid care workers, what meaning does the work have? How do they practice care? Where do these care workers, many of whom are women and disproportionately from minority groups, get their staying power?[9]

Meeting the Staff

Before me is a tribunal of seven women sitting on one side of a long table in a worker's canteen, a place I would come to understand as the "cooler" when stress looms large. There is no hint of shyness on the part of these CNAs and their Charge Nurse—rather, curiosity mixed with suspicion; their eyes burn into mine. My stomach gets queasy. I feel inadequate to the task of convincing them to allow me to live in their world for several hours a day, five days a week. I begin,

> I'm a researcher, and I am very interested in what you do in your work and what the social world of an Alzheimer's Pavilion is like. The best way for me to learn and to understand what you do is to, basically, hang out on the Pavilion.

As the minutes tick by and I explain in more detail my presence in their workplace, the crossed arms and poker faces of the women facing me form a united front. After I finish, there is one question from a CNA who lowers her head and peers under the open table separating me from them. With a sly, mischievous grin on her face, she asks, "You're not thinkin' of wearing those high heel shoes and that outfit down here are ya?" For a split second there is a deafening silence and then everyone, including me, breaks into uproarious laughter. I had just been tested by Licensed Practical Nurse (LPN)[10] Marita Martin and her team of care workers at Starrmount Alzheimer's Pavilion. Needless to say my high heel shoes and professional clothing never saw the light of day again in the Pavilion.

The frontline staff of the Alzheimer's Pavilion have hard lives outside the Pavilion, caring for husbands or children in prison, confronting suicides, surviving on low incomes and dealing with health problems. According to Charge Nurse, Marita Martin, some come from abused backgrounds themselves which, she argues, makes them more sensitive to the residents "because they have lived with pain." The female, African American staff consist of five CNAs and an LPN Mexican American Charge Nurse, a former CNA. All staff have been working on the Pavilion for at least five years and have a high school diploma or General Educational Diploma, except the newest CNA who has been at Starrmount for one year. Most of the Alzheimer's staff had to "learn everything from the beginning" as founder of the Pavilion, RN[11] Elaine Pressley put it.

Women of Color in a World Apart follows the lives of staff and residents over a year and a half as CNAs defend and maintain their workplace culture, carving out a different model of care in resistance[12] to the medical model.

Notes

1 All staff and resident names as well as the name of the research site in this study are pseudonyms. Initially, I introduce residents using their full names and thereafter refer to them as they were addressed on the Pavilion, either by their given names or the nicknames that the staff have given them. As I worked on the book, I chose different pseudonyms for CNAs than those used in previously published articles so as to better represent their personalities.

2 Certified Nursing Assistants provide much of the hands-on care in hospitals, nursing homes and other health care facilities. Mostly women of color, these workers live at or just below the poverty line and are placed in a job that in the United States is at the lower end of the occupational ladder in terms of formal skills; however, nursing assistants are closest to the patient, and, to varying degrees, understand and are privy to the intimate lives of their charges. Everett Hughes, "Good People and Dirty Work," *Social Problems* 10 (1) (1962): 3–11, calls such work "dirty work." According to the 2017 report on direct care workers by the *Paraprofessional Healthcare Institute*, almost 20 percent of Nursing Home CNAs live below the poverty line, rely on public benefits and have meager wages. As a society, we do not recognize nor reward this level of essential care work.

3 From a biomedical perspective, Senile Dementia of the Alzheimer's type (SDAT) is a progressive, irreversible, degenerative brain disease, involving a decline in intellectual functioning, memory loss, paranoid thinking and bizarre behavior, Barry Reisberg, *Alzheimer's Disease* (New York: Free Press, 1983). According to the *2017 Alzheimer's Disease Facts and Figures Report*, over 5 million Americans live with Alzheimer's dementia which could increase to 16 million by 2050 at a cost of 1.1 trillion to the nation. At present, more than 15 million Americans provide unpaid care for people with dementia, valued at $230 billion; however, the move to long-term care (nursing home, hospice) is almost inevitable due to the nature of the disease and extreme caregiver burden. The so-called Baby Boom cohort is expected to be a demographic challenge that has the potential to place a significant burden on the health care system as early as 2030 and most certainly by 2050. Moreover, with the demographic explosion in America of the "oldest old" (eighty-five years and beyond), caregiving for aged persons has become an important topic, transforming private struggles into public concerns.

As a nation we are facing what social policy analysts argue is a severe labor shortage of nurses and nursing assistants in both acute hospital care and especially in long-term care now and into the future. Poor working environments within America's health care system have contributed to a high annual turnover rate of nurses and nursing assistants from burnout. The annual average turnover rate for Certified Nursing Assistants is 70 percent. In contrast, five out of six of Starrmount CNAs and the LPN Charge Nurse have been on the Pavilion between five and eight years. This low turnover rate is an unusual feature in such facilities in the United States. Unlike the Starrmount staff, research on causes of nurse's aide turnover in nursing homes indicates lack of teamwork, exclusion from communication processes between CNAs and nurses, and exclusion from interdisciplinary care plan meetings as primary reasons for turnover. See Jane Banaszak-Holl and Marilyn A. Hines, "Factors Associated with Nursing Home Staff Turnover," *Gerontologist* 36 (August 1996): 512–517; Patricia Parmelee, Mary Laszio and Jo Taylor, "Perceived Barriers to Effective Job Performance Among Nursing Assistants in Long-term Care," *Journal of the American Medical Directors Association* 10 (October 2009): 559–556. Also, Connie Madden et al., "Rules of Performance in the Nursing Home: A Grounded Theory of Nurse-CNA Communication," *Geriatric Nursing* 38 (2017): 378–384.

4 Starrmount Geriatric Center is a nonprofit, private multi-care facility with independent living apartments and an intermediate and skilled nursing care center located in a mid-western city. The Helen Wise Alzheimer's Pavilion is part of Starrmount with a staff of five CNAs who are African American, and a Mexican American licensed practical nurse (LPN) as the charge nurse of the Alzheimer's Pavilion. An activities worker provides regular structured activities for the residents, which range from drawing/painting to quizzes, to sing-alongs, to attending events upstairs in the convocation room. The Pavilion has a city-wide "reputation of being the best." They are always getting calls and have a two-year waiting list. Peripheral staff connected to the Pavilion are an RN Head Nurse, a Director of Nursing and a Social Service Worker. All residents in the first and second level units are ambulatory while the third unit is for non-ambulatory residents with dementia.

5 The social science book-length literature on nursing assistants' labor is sparse. Those studies that had an impact on this study are Jaber F. Gubrium, *Living and Dying at Murray Manor* (New York: St. Martin's Press, 1975), an ethnographic classic revealing detail on the day-to-day workings of the nursing home. He discloses the adversarial relationship

between staff and residents and the daily grind of what he calls "bed and body work" where lower level nurse's aides are paid a pittance and carry out their work on the aged as objects; Timothy Diamond, *Making Gray Gold: Narratives of Nursing Home Care* (Chicago, IL and London: University of Chicago Press, 1992); and, Nancy Foner, *The Caregiving Dilemma: Work in an American Nursing Home* (Berkeley, CA: University of California Press, 1995). Jay Gubrium has contributed a large body of work on the social meanings of Alzheimer's disease: Jay Gubrium, *Oldtimers and Alzheimers: The Descriptive Organization of Senility* (Greenwich, CT: JAI Press, 1986), which provides important insight from his research in an Alzheimer's day hospital. In his article, "The Social Preservation of Mind: The Alzheimer's Disease Experience," *Symbolic Interaction* 9 (1986): 37–51, Gubrium demonstrates the importance of the social environment surrounding the person with Alzheimer's disease in preserving mind, and focuses on the use of language and social meanings in a later article, Jaber Gubrium and Robert Lynott, "Measurement and the Interpretation of Burden in the Alzheimer's Disease Experience," *Journal of Aging Studies* 1 (1987): 265–285. The path-breaking social-psychological work of the late Tom Kitwood, *Dementia Reconsidered: The Person Comes First* (Buckingham: Open University Press, 1997) was an early inspiration.

Other social science studies, which provide a *context* for mine, are ethnographies in the 1980s that produced critical analysis of seemingly entrenched, bleak conditions within U.S. nursing homes, for example, Bruce Vladeck, *Unloving Care: The Nursing Home Tragedy* (New York: Basic Books, 1980), which urged reform measures culminating in the National Institute of Medicine's 1986 report, *Improving the Quality of Care in Nursing Homes.* Later studies in the 1980s revealed a number of institutional constraints within nursing homes that mitigate the quality of care, namely, poor wages and understaffing, very high turnover rates, burnout of nursing personnel (particularly frontline workers such as CNAs) and excessive paperwork, for example, Renée Shield, *Uneasy Endings: Daily Life in an American Nursing Home* (Ithaca, NY: Cornell University Press, 1988); and Jeanie Kayser-Jones, *Old, Alone and Neglected* (Berkeley, CA: University of California Press, 1981), who describes aides as blatantly physically abusive in the form of taking out personal problems on patients. CNAs are described as insensitive, victimizing, authoritative, disrespectful and infantilizing in their treatment of elderly patients. In the 1990s, social science researchers began to focus on the consequences of social structure on staff and patient behavior which revealed a more complex, nuanced picture of CNAs' care work. Certified Nursing Assistants employ more skills in their work as frontline caregivers within long-term care institutions than previously documented: Jay Savishinsky, *The Ends of Time: Life and Work in a Nursing Home* (New York: Bergin and Garvey, 1991); Timothy Diamond, *Making Gray Gold* (Chicago, IL: University of Chicago Press, 1992); Nancy Foner, *The Caregiving Dilemma: Work in an American Nursing Home* (Berkeley, CA: University of California Press, 1995); Neil Henderson and Maria Vesperi (eds), *The Culture of Long Term Care: Nursing Home Ethnography* (Westport, CT: Praeger, 1995).

Most recently, Jason Rodriquez's book, *Labors of Love: Nursing Homes and the Structures of Care Work* (New York: New York University Press, 2014), concentrates on nursing home managers, emotional labor and organizational structures of a for-profit and a nonprofit nursing home. I engage with Rodriquez's book in his discussion of emotional care.

6 This book builds on the classic work of Timothy Diamond, *Making Gray Gold: Narratives of Nursing Home Care* (Chicago, IL: University of Chicago Press, 1992) in his call for

a potentially transformative "vocabulary of care" based on CNA knowledge and on the classic work of Nancy Foner, *The Caregiving Dilemma: Work in an American Nursing Home* (Berkeley, CA: University of California Press, 1995) in her critical question, "How might autonomy for CNAs help, rather than hurt patient care?" (The word, autonomy, has its origins in Greek language and culture. Avrovouia, the Greek word for autonomy, means having or making one's own laws and having independence. As it is used here, autonomy is best understood as self-determination and can take different forms in the world of the Pavilion.)

To date, there has been no social science book-length, systematic investigation of these crucial issues raised by Diamond and Foner. The book breaks new ground and fills this gap. For a year and a half I conducted participant observation in Starrmount Pavilion along with intensive interviewing of Certified Nursing Assistants, the Charge Nurse and the Director of Nursing in the latter 1990s. I set out to observe and engage the residents in conversation as they contributed to the construction of care work. As well, I interviewed family members so that I might analyze the public and private domains of care as they intersect. The data were generated from twenty-six residents, intensive interviews with forty-one staff and family members and health diaries kept by three CNAs. Observations were continuous and multiple over an extended period, in a variety of situations, at varying times. I set out to construct a sequential process in my participant observation and intensive interviewing that commenced with those residents who had the least power through circumstances or illness. Interpretation grounded securely in the empirical world provides a fresh perspective on paid care work. I observed and talked with the CNAs and the LPN Charge Nurse over a long period of time, gaining their trust and becoming a part of their world. "Is there anything exciting going on here today?" I would ask the residents as I surveyed the family room for a place to sit that felt right for that day. Sometimes I would sit near the nurse's alcove amongst the residents in one of the low, sturdy rocking chairs in the sitting group. My choice of seats was mostly random to observe and talk with those who had the least amount of power in the setting. I could always keep an eye out for what was happening with the CNAs near me while devoting my attention to residents and resident–staff interaction. I conducted approximately four to five hours of observation daily, on an average of four days a week (7:00 am to 3:00 pm) I varied the times I entered and left the site to get an immediate and different impression from the very first moment I stepped on the Pavilion.

I spent many hours conducting open-ended, in-depth interviews resulting in a large amount of narrative that revealed the individual perspective and served as a point of contrast or corroboration of material garnered from observation. Tape-recorded interviews with a staff member averaged five to nine hours each and two to three hours each with family members, yielding 1,422 pages of transcript. At first, staff struggled to give voice to something they had never articulated—the meaning and conditions of their work. Speaking through the medium of the interview, the workers confronted the challenge of giving words to a knowledge that seems to defy words and their ability to "read" what appears as unintelligible in the residents. Their reflections hold both wonder as awe and wonder-ing as cognitive process. Through strategic probing, staff became able to articulate what they know and how they feel but had never been asked to reveal in depth and detail. My primary methodological sources for the research come from the writings of John and Lyn Lofland, *Analyzing Social Settings* (Boston, MA: Cengage, 1994); James Spradley, *The Ethnographic Interview* (Chicago,

IL: Holt, Rinehart and Winston, 1979); James Spradley, *Participant Observation* (Chicago, IL: Holt, Rinehart and Winston, 1980); Elliot G. Mishler, *Research Interviewing: Context and Narrative* (Cambridge, MA: Harvard University Press, 1986); Clifford Geertz, *Local Knowledge: Further Essays in Interpretive Anthropology* (New York: Basic Books, 1983); and Robert Emerson, Rachel Fretz and Linda Shaw, *Writing Ethnographic Fieldnotes* (Chicago, IL: University of Chicago Press, 2011).

7 This is a book about the social construction of paid care work within an institutional setting. I define paid care as both a *practice (labor)* and a *relation* that are inextricably bound. As a practice, paid care work in the health care field is instrumental and involves assisting persons with the activities of daily living (dressing, grooming, feeding, bathing, toileting, administering medications). As a relation, I view care work as emotional, as the mode or kind of connection between one person and another or others. Such a perspective is important because it not only includes the idea of care as a functional duty that one is paid to do but also investigates how and where the relation of care ("being" as a care worker) is constructed, negotiated, contested, frustrated and threatened. While it is possible to use the concept of relationship, I choose to use relation because it is precise and without valence. From a feminist standpoint, I do not want to assume that there is an "inherent" disposition, tendency, or inclination to care in a person, particularly in women. I particularly like Diemut Bubeck's work, *Care, Gender and Justice* (Oxford, Clarendon Press, 1995: 129) for its emphasis on the *interactional*, and her subtle distinction of the

> relation aspect of care as the meeting of the needs of one person by another person where face-to-face interaction between carer and cared for is a crucial element of the overall activity and where the need is of such a nature that it cannot possibly be met by the person in need herself.

8 The book challenges the assumptions of the outside world that low-level women workers have only minimal skills, and just put in a day's labor. CNA Justine King's confrontation with the substitute aide is but one of several strategies staff members may use when the moral rights of residents or their own moral rights are threatened. These women are real people acting in real situations who create and react, struggle and fail, initiate and cope as they create an alternative model of care work. There are two overarching themes of the book. First, we examine the various processes that produce meaningfully personal care by CNAs in the kind of nursing home situation that is synonymous with impersonal, non-caring treatment. Justine King's demand for respect is not just lip service to a concept. It is a part of the staff members' ethic of care out of which their work arises. Through her interaction with the substitute aide, Justine constructs one element of care and conveys to an outsider an image of herself and the collective of CNAs. Second, we examine how this care is interactionally produced, what it looks like, and how it is achieved moment to moment in CNA dealings with residents, when they fail and when they succeed in creating a pocket of alternative care work amid the bureaucracy.

My primary theoretical sources for the research are the symbolic interaction/social constructionist perspective, the writings of George Herbert Mead, Herbert Blumer and Erving Goffman. For Mead, *Mind, Self and Society* (Chicago, IL: University of Chicago Press, 1934), both mind and self arise out of the social; self and society are "twin born"; the self is active, not passive; and, experience must be analyzed from the "standpoint of communication (through the use of symbols) as essential to the social order." Blumer, *Symbolic Interaction: Perspective and* Method (Oakland, CA: University of California Press, 1986: 180), states:

> The term "symbolic interactionism" refers … to the peculiar and distinctive character of interaction as it takes place between human beings. The peculiarity consists in the fact that human beings interpret or "define" each other's actions instead of merely reacting to each other's actions. Their "response" is not made directly to the actions of one another but instead based on the meaning which they attach to such actions. Thus, human interaction is mediated by the use of symbols, by interpretation, or by ascertaining the meaning of one another's actions.

Also, Goffman's analysis of varied social situations from a symbolic interactionist position, in particular, *Asylums* (New York: Anchor, 1961) and "The Insanity of Place," *Psychiatry: Journal for the Study of Interpersonal Processes*, vol XXXII (1969): 362, 366, provided important sources.

9 What do these workers, whom many would think dislike their jobs, find meaningful in their work? More importantly, how does the construction of work as meaningful come about? CNAs live in a world of *circumscribed opportunities* so that their choices about work are constrained. As working-class black women, the CNAs have been curtailed in their choice of work through opportunity structures in place in American society. The CNAs bear the weight of responsibility for the care of what some in our society, even some in the geriatric facility itself, call "crazies." How can what many would consider an excessively demanding job be a refuge as well for CNAs?

10 According to the 2010–2011 *Occupational Outlook Handbook,* Bureau of Labor Statistics, a Licensed Practical Nurse (LPN) provides "basic nursing care, must complete a state-approved educational program of a year and must be licensed." LPNs are often supervised by a Registered Nurse (RN) and in turn, supervise CNAs.

11 An RN is a Registered Nurse who has graduated from an accredited nursing program and passed a state board examination, and has been registered and licensed to practice nursing. RNs provide care and serve as supervisors of LPNs and CNAs.

12 This study follows sociologist, Randy Hodson and anthropologist/political scientist, James C. Scott in exploring the multiple ways resistance can be demonstrated by low-level workers in work and social settings such as the Pavilion. Their perspectives are path-breaking in moving beyond the traditional working-class literature which has "focused on blatant, violent acts of sabotage or on a definition of resistance that is highly organized, cooperative, etc. and discards actions that are what Scott calls "garden variety resistance" used by subservient groups: James C. Scott, *Weapons of the Weak: Everyday Forms of Peasant Resistance* (New Haven, CT: Yale University Press, 1987: 292). Randy Hodson, *Dignity at Work* (Cambridge: Cambridge University Press, 2001: 723), argues that "The specific behavioral strategies of resistance used by workers to attain their goals are limited only by their creativity. Worker resistance is often quite subtle in its forms of expression." For more on the construction of resistance, see Randy Hodson and Victor Roscigno, "Worker resistance: An Underdeveloped Concept in the Sociology of Work," *Economic and Industrial Democracy*, 16 (1995): 79–110.

1

IN PLACE ON THE PAVILION

My watch reads 6:40 am. The steps leading into the main lobby of Starrmount Geriatric Center seem higher at this hour as I greet Suzanne at the front desk and sign in. I find it easy to imagine I am in a stately old hotel. The walls of expensive honey brown paneling dressed in plaques convey respectability and a long history. Richly upholstered chairs and traditional sofas dot the perimeter of the expansive lobby. The stillness of the hour is broken by the muffled voices of those opening the gift shop. Waving to Mary who tends the shop, I cross the gleaming parquet floor and head for the stairs to take me down to the Garden Level.

Once on the ground floor, I am taken hostage by the harsh, unforgiving fluorescent lights. I make my way through a narrow corridor of whitewashed cinderblock walls, past the utility and laundry rooms in the lower reaches of social space until I am face-to-face with the Helen Wise Alzheimer's Pavilion.

I do not know the world I am about to enter this day. Negotiating the panel with the code that grants me physical entrance, I hesitate in the transition space between the larger institutional world and the world of the Pavilion. I remember a family member referring to it as the "preparation space," a place for the family to ready themselves and to locate their family member in the distance. This funnel-like passageway allows one to view the goings on before entering the public space that contains a kitchen-dining area, living room, and a small nurse's station. Resident rooms line the right perimeter to complete an L-shaped configuration.

Resident Harriet French sees me and approaches quickly, as I hear the heavy door shut behind me. A wiry woman, her salt and pepper hair tangled, though not fashionably so, she runs, her legs propelling her directly toward me. Without enough arms and understanding to gather her in, I fear she will fall and take me with her, such is her intensity. Harriet is a musician and a former music teacher. With bright eyes and big energy, she greets me though I cannot understand her words. Clad in a red-checkered skirt and red sweater, she has allowed her crisp white blouse to escape her skirt, a hint of the incompleteness of the morning dressing combined with her restlessness and a propensity to disrobe. She grabs my forearm and pulls me toward an imagined destination. The brightness in her eyes turns to unknowable yearning when she looks up at me. As I put my arm around her shoulder I wonder if she has been up all night.

Alighting from the entry, Harriet and I find ourselves in an expansive space with the palest of blue walls. Just as powerfully as she sought me out, Harriet turns away and clasps arms with her friend, Susan. Bodies moving in tandem, they walk away chattering to one another. To my left, natural light pours through sliding glass doors looking out onto an enclosed courtyard, a place affording protection and the potential for pleasure. Residents may amble through quadrants of grass and onto walkways lined with bright pink and white blooms, the last fruits of an Indian summer. In the center is a small fountain, pleasing in its simplicity. Yet, there is no mistaking this courtyard to be private. When Harriet and the other residents walk into the garden they can be watched because the courtyard is encircled by three floors of the institution. The purpose of the building design is to provide visual pleasure but also to provide ample opportunity for surveillance of residents. A comparison with the Panopticon[1] is not out of the question.

I walk past the dining area, which consists of six tables, usually in two rows, end to end. If not aesthetically pleasing, it is nonetheless functional and remarkably clean given its multipurpose use. Just ahead is the residents' sitting area—a square enclosed by chairs and a television in one corner, an island of blue carpet on a sea of white linoleum. Artwork on a pillar separating the sitting room from the dining areas reminds me of residents gathering to draw with the art therapist on Monday and Thursday mornings. My eyes travel past the large fish tank to the nurses' station, an alcove tucked away at the farthest point from the entrance, directly across from the sitting area.

Only a few residents are stirring, either the early risers or those who stayed up all night. Miss Ava Reynolds is one of the all-nighters who may remain awake for forty-eight hours after which she collapses and sleeps "like the dead" for a day. The lighting is mellow and sounds are muted with only a hint of activity behind residents' doors. Martin Lovett, a small, gentle man given to occasional emotional outbursts, is sitting on the blue sofa snoozing. He was in the "big time" in one of the largest cities in the U.S. as a "crackerjack" newscaster, according to his son who is so stunned by his father's demise he cannot come to see him. The son fears visiting with his father will be so emotionally upsetting that he cannot do his work as a newspaper reporter.

Over my right shoulder comes wafting, "One, two, three, out goes she into the deep blue sea … Softball seven eleven." Marge Jacobs dances up to me, pausing in her rhyming to respond to my "Good Morning to you." She continues to move in place, full of energy, expectant, trying to find the words to say what's on her mind and "doing her little dance" as one CNA calls it. Her legs and head are perfectly synchronized in an up and down motion, jam-packed with bursts of energy. Marge's presence is electric. I walk back through the sitting area where residents Boris Randolph and David Hogan are on the couch. Mr. Randolph wears his customary hat and jacket and David Hogan sports a colorful long-sleeve shirt. I wave and they wave back.

On this autumn day I look out through the large window wall that frames the courtyard and notice the leaves on the tree in the center seem to have changed color overnight. Resident Paulina Creed is standing next to the sliding glass doors, peering out. Her hands are clasped behind her back in a familiar pose, a little bun poised atop her head, a diminutive, yet hardy figure. She gazes upward at the trees. I walk over:

ANNE: Anything exciting going on here this morning?
PAULINA: Well no, but it's fun.
ANNE: What did you do that was fun?
PAULINA: Well, going out, sitting under the trees, looking at the leaves, watching the birds, and so forth.
ANNE: Did you notice that the leaves are turning a color?
PAULINA: Oh, I wondered … I think it's nice that it turned that color. It probably amuses the tree that way too.
ANNE: (Hesitating to catch my breath at the cleverness of her response) That's an interesting observation. We had a couple of cold nights last week.
PAULINA: Ohhhhhh … (raising her voice slightly in recognition) Well, you mean … ah … that they're ah … losing their ability to produce things?
ANNE: Right. To produce chlorophyll that makes the leaf green.
PAULINA: (With earnest concern) Well, is there anything we can do about it?
ANNE: Don't think so … but they'll come back next year.
Paulina nods.

In the distance, Charge Nurse Marita and her team of five Certified Nursing Assistants are gathering in the cubby hole that is the nurses' station.

Marita's Leadership

LPN Marita Martin lives so near Starrmount Geriatric that she can round the corner from her little house at the end of a cul-de-sac in a working-class neighborhood, shoot across a busy city street, and be there. According to Charge Nurse Marita, in the world of the Helen Wise Alzheimer's Pavilion, "you have to leave your normal self behind when you walk through the doors." Marita, who comes out of a background of poverty, sets the tone in the Pavilion. As leader, she is wise and passionate, and prides herself on being attuned to the individual sensibilities of frail residents. Marita worked in a psychiatric setting as a frontline worker before coming to Starrmount and has a learned psychological acumen. All of "her girls," as she calls them, respect her a great deal even though she gets mad at them sometimes for "sitting around" when they could be thinking of things to do. She tries to build resident morale and works hard at it.

Marita is informed by logic but also sensibility. Her care comes not from a technique that is applied to human objects but from a reservoir within. She is overworked and is a poet of sorts. Marita gave me several of her poems in which she struggles to find and convey a rhythm of effective communication with residents. At any point in the day, she may let down her hair and enfold the residents in spontaneous dancing and singing. She is full of pride for her Mexican heritage but critical of herself for what she thinks are her failures. Her vicarious feelings of pain and questioning are part of a meshing of self-analysis and resident analysis. She has a desire to preserve the dignity of the residents, to have them considered fully "human, inside and outside of the Pavilion."

CNAs settle in for the morning meeting. Some bodies are large, some are small and space in the alcove is at a premium as they take their place on top of desks, leaning against the file cabinets, shoulder-to-shoulder and hip-to-hip. These women know one another on and off the job. At 7:00 am, yawns punctuate tales of lost sleep and morning migraines but soon give way to figuring out Miss Ava's morning routine, letting "Boots" (Verna) and Emma sleep-in as an experiment, and collective groaning at medicine choices that may cause Henrietta Stein's trails of "dreaded" diarrhea. Strong-willed and intelligent, Henrietta tests the mettle of the staff. With a gleam in her eye, CNA Arnella Jackson comments, "I think she does it on purpose, I do, I really do." Several nod in agreement but try to pass it off good-naturedly.

Arnella's Insights

Arnella Jackson's insights come from seven years of observation on the Pavilion. Arnella is characterized by Marita as "the organizer. She can get things done. If she says she is going to do it, she does it. She doesn't procrastinate." Arnella has a family to whom she can talk about her work and let off steam. On the one hand she likens the Alzheimer's residents to "children that like to get your attention and have their own little way of getting it." On the other hand, she emphasizes, "They are not children and we don't treat them as children."

Arnella recognizes many sides of resident behavior and is adept at using metaphors to describe such behavior:

> I hate to compare it to this but it's like when it's a full moon and the werewolf gets loose and he just goes into a frenzy. Some residents are like that in the afternoon. Some of them become verbally abusive, some of them become physically abusive.

She understands because her grandmother was diagnosed with probable Alzheimer's disease.

As I watch Arnella throughout her day's work, she is precise and thorough, moving rhythmically and expeditiously throughout the space. She likes to bring order to situations and laser-like shoots to the source to quell the disorder. The emotional aspect of her work and the amount of patience she must have with the residents are critical elements in her care. When I asked her how many eyes and ears it takes to work in this place, she answered, "Thousands." She believes she has an ability to intuit what is "going on" with a resident or with a team member. There are times when she is feeling at the end of her rope and as she relates, "I must go to the cooler, smoke a cigarette, and give myself time to come back to my senses."

Arnella has a sly sense of humor and a steady, usually even temperament; however, she can become very angry when giving me examples of people who come to the Pavilion and disrespect residents. She is dedicated to providing equal treatment to the residents and not "neglecting" anyone.

Everything is relaxed, familiar as the morning meeting begins with Marita perched atop the desk console. "With regard to Ruby, just let her sleep until she gets tired of it." Resident Ruby Klein has been on the mend from an accident where she fell and broke her pelvis. She is making progress, but slowly. At times, she is disheartened by not being able to walk and by the pain. "Also, let Mary sleep later if she wants," Marita continues.

> We do have to change that mattress. It smells so bad. And Barbara Cole is on a special "cal" (calorie) sheet now because she's lost too much weight. Well, you know she's always been a little eater anyway. I tried to explain that to Susan (the head of dietary) but they still have to put the weight down so that State (nursing home regulators) will see that we're trying to do something. We may want to start her on Great Shakes and just give her that. Why don't we give it to her at mealtime and in-between and see what happens.

Peering over her glasses, CNA Arnella asks Marita Martin a question that is on everyone's mind.

"The Great Shakes don't cause diarrhea, do they?"

At this point the rest of the CNAs are chuckling, making faces and gagging.

"I wondered why you were staring at me," Marita says laughingly.

"Again, I say, does it cause diarrhea?" Arnella quips, barely suppressing her laugh.

"Yes it does."

In unison the CNAs groan, "Ohhhhhhh …"

"Marie had 'em yesterday and she made a big mess," offers CNA Carma Lee. "She cussed me out yesterday. I tell you I put a diaper on her on Tuesday and it came out, and it wasn't on her diaper anywhere. It was *ev-v-erywhere*" (chuckling).

Carma Lee's "Mental Work"

CNA Carma Lee is a quiet but determined person who rises to the challenges when carrying out her duties with the residents. She focuses on the "self-esteem" of a resident and what she thinks she can do to sustain that. Carma Lee worked with paraplegics, the disabled and people with Down Syndrome before the Starrmount Alzheimer's Pavilion. She chose this work because she enjoys helping people. Several times, she has been the recipient of "employee of the month," which covers all floors of Starrmount. For Carma Lee, it is not nearly enough to enter a comment on the chart such as "patient no longer cares about being clean, doesn't talk very much" because this condition may be an indication of the loss of self-esteem, which is not recorded. Psychologically oriented, Carma tries to keep in mind that "people want you to show them the same respect even if they are sick." She believes the moods of the staff affect the residents and "One can get into the habit of not caring. It's not the most highest paying job in the world and your own self-esteem can get to be very low. You have to bring yourself up."

Carma Lee views the bed and body work as secondary to the mental work, residents' feelings being "number one" for her. She is fiercely protective of the residents and committed to upholding their rights. When she gets too stressed out and the residents get on her nerves, she "pictures herself in the situation and that they're sick and it's part of the sickness, not the person." She has deep confidence in her religious beliefs and when asked how she got through the first weeks on the Pavilion, she said, "A lot of times, believe me, it was a lot of prayer and long suffering. Physically, I had it made, but just mentally I said, 'Oh boy.'" She can become weary and blue but explains how the residents form a "buddy system" very much like a community which "really encouraged" her to stay in the job. According to Marita Martin, "Carma Lee and Chevelle are the ones that keep us on the level of we're humans. We have feelings. We have emotions. They're kind of like the mother, the mothers that you go to for nurturing."

As the meeting continues, CNAs Justine and Arnella hear resident Ruby calling from her room.

"Ooooops, Ruby's up."

They look at each other.

"That's early for Ruby," they say almost in unison.

"She's soooo sleepy," Arnella says. "I thought she'd be in bed until about 10:30. Let me go get her because she'll be upset."

"Say, Marita, when did Boris (a recently hospitalized resident) go out?" Justine asks.

"He was real cooperative. We called the ambulance."

"But I thought he wasn't to go."

"OK. Here's what happened. Judy (another LPN) came over after we left for the day and his leg was badly swollen," Marita explains.

"I really wonder if the last time he was in there (the hospital) that was the problem and they couldn't find anything." Justine's voice rises, "And we kept saying and kept saying ... Why didn't they keep him? (shaking her head). I bet you anything that's what was wrong then. He developed a real redness on the foot and it was real warm."

"I know, Justine," responds Marita in a tone of resignation. "Well, he's back in his room now so we can see him later. Whoever has Marge, we can't get her up until I get that x-ray."

"If she goes to therapy she'll be like Ruby," Justine says. "She'll snap on back. I want her back (a silence) ... I want her back ... Marita ..."

"I do too." "Oh, Catherine's tennis shoes are in the top drawer. I wish we did have some puffed wheat for the residents. They keep bringing rice krispies." "Maybe, I just need to get over there (to dietary) and talk to some people," Justine says in a defiant tone.

Justine's "Power and Passion"

CNA Justine King is a powerful black woman who says what she means and means what she says. She is bold and a bit daunting to strangers. When I first met her, she intimidated me; for the first six months of observation, I felt I was a target of her gaze. When my "probation period" was over and we made it to common ground I found out she *was* watching *me* as I watched *them*. Justine explained she wanted to "see how I treated the residents." Needless to say I was relieved that I had passed the test. Justine is one on whom nothing is lost. For me, there was no question that hers was the most important trust I must earn.

Justine is fiercely territorial, a leader, and a rebel. She consistently uses her analytical abilities to learn from the residents and "understand where they are coming from." Justine has killer migraines and multiple strains on her from her family situation. Her son is in and out of jail and she has the care of her "grandbaby" whom she thinks about "all the time she is not thinking about one of the residents." She and Arnella have a peer understanding as they communicate tacitly as well as explicitly throughout the day. Sometimes Justine is quick to anger and proud of what she and the others do on the Pavilion and does not hesitate to let the novice know it. Her heart is big and her fuse short when it comes to protecting the residents from humiliation or verbal abuse by "outsiders." Marita says Justine "represents the strength that is within the group. She can keep us together when we fall apart. She always has something good to say, positive."

On the Pavilion, residents make racist remarks. While she doesn't overtly fight back Justine maintains an inner boiling point with one resident in particular. She is both patient and petulant and is drawn to residents who she calls "loud." "I like to see my residents strong, with just the right touch of being uppity," she says, a trait she seems fond of in herself as well.

At this moment, someone from dietary comes over and says they will guarantee puffed wheat by the end of the week. Justine and the other CNAs spar with her in good humor and ask if they can have that in writing.

MARITA: As for Miss Ava, test the waters first and let her sleep until 9:30–10:00. Medicine is the problem. I don't want my residents doped up and ready to fall asleep all the time. And Arnella, you know when you went in there and let Mary sleep late … well … she was so much better.

ARNELLA: Yeh, she was soooo happy. Because when I got her up she was ready to get up. She drank her juice and ate a little bit of cereal. Getting Boots up, I'm gonna need some help.

CHEVELLE: I'll be there.

Chevelle's Humanity

Chevelle Morris is demure and sweet with the residents. She notices the traits in residents that speak to her of what she calls their "inner being." Chevelle describes herself as a person who "fits in" and "mostly goes along with everything," although this does not mean she doesn't have firm positions on care and a moral code. She likes talking to the residents; for her, many had an "important life. They did something worthwhile and they just get old." Chevelle has a hearty laugh that is infectious. She talks about the stress that occurs on the Pavilion and how she handles it. On the one hand, Chevelle says that she tries "not to get too involved. I can't do that." Getting too involved means for her, "getting too close to the residents. That can easily happen. I try not to do that because I want to be okay." She has gotten more involved and she "felt kinda sad. I didn't like feeling like that all the time so I just take care of them the best I can and that's the way I leave it."

Chevelle wants to learn more about the disease, "to advance because there is always something you can learn about it." In a place where the individuality of residents is ever-present in the minds of the CNAs, she enjoys expressions of residents. One of her favorite phrases is "Their faces just light up" when residents see their spouse come into the Pavilion. She stays on "pins and needles" a lot of the time because of the intermittent flare-ups and inconsistent behavior of some residents.

> They may cuss you out one minute and hug you the next. You have to shift your responses all during the day. It's not an easy thing to deal with these people. You have to deal with so much dealing with the different levels of the residents.

She feels that working on the Pavilion, however, is right for her because she likes to "see some of the residents meet their little freedom." Chevelle has a sense of humor that keeps her afloat during the day. In conversation one day, Chevelle tells me that it is important for the CNAs to take breaks and says, "Every so often I go to the non-smoking room and drink a pop or something. Just relax and then go back. It helps. Fifteen minutes helps a lot." I ask her, "Do you do any talking to yourself during that time?" "No," she says emphatically. Instantly we catch each other's eye, realize the double meaning, and burst into laughter.

Looking over the residents' charts, Arnella, Chevelle, Carma Lee, Glenda and Justine read the night shift's entries for each of their charges. The categories delimit the range of categories with the body writ large: body temperature, pulse rate, blood pressure and respiratory rate, weight, bladder and bowel routines, bathing, bed-making, restraint sheet, eating habits, weight, medication regime, sleeping patterns. The following questions are important for change in level-of-care determination: does the patient still feed him/herself? Is the patient continent or incontinent? Incontinent of bowels or bladder? Does the patient put on his/her own shoes? Does he/she recognize you? Does he/she know your name? What is written in the chart becomes more "real" than what happens in the lifeworld[2] of the residents.

The CNAs' routine is familiar—getting prepped for the expected while, in body and mind, braced for the unexpected in the hours to come until their shift is officially over at 3:00 pm. As the group breaks up and heads out into the world of the residents, Justine calls to Joy Donaldson, a well-dressed former housewife who recently came to the Pavilion, loses her cherished "pocketbook" every few minutes, and longs to "go home" to her family. "Hey girl, hey girl how you doin'? You want some coffee?"

"It's Like Steppin' Through Saran Wrap"

The big wall clock chimes 8:00 am when LPN Marita Martin calls me to the family room. She is transfixed by a group of residents. She moves her eyes across the scene like a searchlight and scrutinizes every movement

"Do you sense anything coming from that part of the room?" she asks. She points to the area where several residents are sitting. Before I can respond, she continues,

> There's an aura. It's an invisible presence (she laughs nervously). I don't want you to think I'm crazy. It was centered around that area there. I was waiting for someone else to get up and do something. I thought something's about to happen and I don't know what it is. Well, after Harriet had slapped Evelyn, that's when I felt it even more. It was there in the morning but a low-key presence at that time. Then throughout the day things just started to unravel and everyone was restless, angry. They were saying "shut up, go to hell" and all that. It was totally weird. Louisa is a prime example. I know when she is ready to blow up and I tell the girls to watch her closer because she can hit on people.

"What makes you think she will do that," I ask.

"Nothing I can put into words. It's just that I have that sense. Sometimes it scares me. Sometimes I sense things with the girls and something is there."

"Does this have both negative and positive outcomes?"

"Yeh. I try to practice it but I'm scared to go into it in depth. Sometimes I will feel this and that's exactly what happens. I can sense the negative more than the positive."

Instead of a taken-for-granted reality, "shifting realities" of the resident must be caught, entered and traversed. As one CNA remarked, "Every day is a surprise, unpredictable. I don't know what to expect when I get here." Therefore, to communicate with individual residents, meaning must be constructed continuously.

In the following description, Marita hears herself giving voice to "going into the zone," the experience of being in a different reality, what the CNAs call "the resident's world."

> MARITA: Right now, thinking about it, you know what it reminds me of? A piece of saran wrap … that you step into but you don't breathe the same air. This may sound nuts to you, I know. When you sit, and whatever the subject matter is, you live there for that moment. When that moment is gone you have to step back through the saran wrap, which is a little more difficult because I like it. Sometimes I do not want to come out of that world. It scares me. The girls (CNAs) feel this way but don't know how to express it. They're comfortable in it. They can answer residents. They can be with them in the moment.[3]

I can attest to what Marita Martin tries to convey, a phenomenon that scholars refer to as a "finite province of meaning." One afternoon, I returned from a stroll with resident Boris Randolph during which I was intensely listening. All of a sudden I am startled by the sound of my name and turn to see a familiar face. The voice belongs to Starrmount CEO John Greenberg who smiles and extends his hand for me to shake. He introduces me to someone from the Alzheimer's Disease Center at the nearby university. I am so disoriented from what Marita might call going into the zone with Boris Randolph that I fumble for words. "So … you're being shown around," I say to the visitor. John Greenberg responds, "I told her you're doing research on the Pavilion." "Yyy-es," I say. John continues, "You are kind of looking at the residents and the staff, how they interact with each other? Sort of along those lines." Again, I murmur, "Yes," accompanied by a nod. "I'm finding I have to carry a tape recorder around with me to catch everything that is going on." "I'll just *bet* you do," Greenberg says, laughing in a manner that presumes we have a shared meaning. When I return to Mr. Randolph, I comprehend how confused I feel and what Marita is trying to find the words to express. The staff speak of it as "going into the zone."

Some version of this scene is repeated countless times within total institutions[4] such as nursing homes and medical facilities across the country as frontline workers prepare for their morning rounds. In nursing homes, care workers attend to the actions of their residents, learn what to expect and gauge how individual residents perceive the surrounding world and their place in it. Care workers share this knowledge with each other, producing a set of shared meanings regarding who each resident is, that is, resident identities, and eventually an ordered set of relations for the setting as well as for each other. The CNAs at Alzheimer's Pavilion at Starrmount describe the outcome as what they believe to be their "different" world of care.[5]

Notes

1 Jeremy Bentham, *The Panopticon Writings*, ed. Miran Bozovic (London: Verso, 1995: 29), an eighteenth century English social philosopher and social theorist, conceived of and constructed a

> Panopticon or inspection house containing a new principle of construction applicable to any sort of establishment in which persons of any description are to be kept under inspection. The circular structure was designed so that those being observed would be unable to tell whether they were being watched.

2 From a sociological perspective, the life world is life as experienced by persons together – the world of everyday life. Alfred Schutz, *The Phenomenology of the Social World* (Evanston, IL: Northwestern University Press, 1970).

3 Peter Berger and Thomas Luckmann, *The Social Construction of Reality: A Treatise in the Sociology of Knowledge* (New York: Anchor Press, 1967: 21, 23, 25, 26), discuss what they call the "reality of everyday life" that we all live in. It is normal and self-evident.

> The reality of everyday life presents itself as … a world that I share with others. I know that the world of everyday life is as real to others as it is to myself. I cannot exist in everyday life without continually interacting and communicating with others.

The interpersonal context in which the CNAs glean their knowledge of the residents and practice their care work is more akin to what Berger and Luckmann call a "finite reality marked by circumscribed meanings and modes of experience." There is a "jolt" when one leaves the finite province of meaning and re-enters the reality of everyday life. They use an analogy from the theatre for illustration:

> The transition between realities is marked by the rising and falling of the curtain. As the curtain rises the spectator is transported to another world with its own meanings and an order that may or may not have much to do with the order of everyday life. As the curtain falls, the spectator "returns to reality," that is to the paramount reality of everyday life, by comparison with which the reality presented on the stage now appears tenuous and ephemeral.

Marita's metaphorical use of saran wrap, through which one can see the reality of everyday life, ends up being her vivid way of capturing the reality of everyday life, still retaining its paramount status even as she goes into the resident's "finite province of meaning." In contrast to Berger and Luckmann's depiction, however, there are shifting realities implied in the finite province of meaning that Marita talks about. In other words, while the province is finite in relation to the reality of everyday life, it contains within it, multiple meanings, realities, places, and time frames of the resident. Her comments extend this knowledge to the collective, to the staff as a whole. With a boldness mixed with temerity, Marita Martin speaks of the encapsulating quality of being in a finite province of meaning with the resident. She expresses a compelling, almost irresistible desire, to "not come out of this world." She elaborates:

> This sounds so crazy. I've never voiced it. It sounds nuts to me. I know we all have different personalities. I've had enough psych but when I verbalize it, it sounds mad. And as God as my witness, may he strike me dead if I'm lying to you, sometimes I do not want to come out of that world. It scares me as I think about it because it is the first time I've articulated it.

The staff have more control, more respect, more dignity in the Pavilion than "out there" in the world. The desirability of this world is probably elevated to some extent because of the circumstances most staff face on the outside. But, inside the Pavilion, they can participate in creating the world in which they want to live.

4 In his ethnography of a mental hospital, Erving Goffman, *Asylums* (New York: The Free Press, 1961) details the nature of what he calls the "total institution" where all the activities of daily life are taken care of in one place, inmates (patients) are socially controlled by dehumanizing treatment, and there is a split between staff and patients. He gives us a first-hand account of the struggle of the patient self to survive as it is stripped of individuality and dignity, finally to be found residing only in the "crevices of the institutional structure." Nursing Homes in the United States resemble the total institution.

5 While making a few appearances in the book, Diane Morgan, Starrmount CNA activities assistant, and CNA Glenda Johns were not interviewed in depth and profiled. Glenda is a new member of Marita's team of five. Diane rotates on several floors of the nursing home and is not a regular on the Starrmount Pavilion.

2

EVERYDAY AMBIENCE AND CONFLICTS

> You know, it isn't an easy thing to deal with these people. Miss Ava … you don't know what she will do. It's stressful. What do you do now?
>
> —*CNA Chevelle*

With charts in hand, CNAs go in and out of resident rooms not with a bustle but on tip-toe to see who is awake. The mumbling of voices behind half-closed doors crescendos into decipherable exchanges between residents and CNAs. The morning's elemental tasks of toileting, dressing, grooming, changing linens, and bed and body[1] work begin; however, those residents who have an all-nighter's mood may refuse a change of clothes.

"I'm going to see how Ruby's doin,'" Carma Lee calls to Arnella. Ruby Klein likes to sleep late but this morning she is calling out, a sign of "trouble" if Carma Lee cannot get to her before Ruby gets upset. The CNAs disperse for the morning rounds with what Glenda calls their "assignments," five to six residents each weekday. Much of the time the CNAs will not wake Ruby before 10:00 am because as Arnella tells me, "She will get agitated if you go ahead and wake her up." Timing is important in very different ways for different residents. In Ruby's case, it's the difference between a crying outburst and a calmer morning. Ruby is most happy when Carma Lee has time to dress her in her beautiful robe so she can be "Miss Vogue," as the CNAs call her. Then Ruby floats into the dining room on Carma's arm.

Eighty-one-year-old Ruby needs a lot of help in keeping "her self-esteem up" according to Carma Lee who knows her well. Ruby's husband died when she was 66. According to CNA Diane, "Ruby just picked up and took over the family furniture business where she had 'worked retail' ever since she dropped out of school in the 10th grade. Ruby was always on the go, always busy, always a take-charge person," qualities Diane thinks contribute to Ruby's feistiness. "She's just so tiny and she'll stand up and tell somebody off and say 'Get over there and sit down.'" Ever since being diagnosed with probable Alzheimer's disease five years ago, Ruby relies on her nephew to visit and take care of finances.

As we continue to talk, Edna Feldman strides from her room with a skimpy sweatshirt on, no pants, a shirt tied around her neck and one shoe covering part of her right foot. "Come on Edna, let's go put some clothes on," Arnella says. "Don't touch me, everybody hates me," Edna yells. Arnella walks her back to her room and leaves the door open long enough for me to see Arnella and Chevelle attempting to dress Edna with CNA Justine standing nearby. "Come on Edna, it's not gonna hurt. I promise," Chevelle says in a soft voice. All the while Chevelle is holding onto Edna's arms. "It hurts, oh it's awful," Edna shouts. While Arnella is trying to get pants on her she breaks free for an instant and waves her arms uncontrollably before Chevelle uses her strength to bring Edna's arms down to her side so that Arnella can dress her. Edna is screaming at the top of her lungs.

Right at that moment, Louis Feldman, her husband, walks through the entrance of the Pavilion and rushes toward the room. "Please wait out here, Mr. Feldman, until we can get her dressed," Arnella says. "What's happening? I have a right to see her, you bet I do," he says. "Please let us just get her clothes on her," Chevelle says. With that, Arnella turns and shuts the door behind her. Feldman slaps his hand against the side of his leg. His face is frozen in anger. Carma Lee comes over to comfort him but he waves her away as he paces in front of the door. Several minutes later, Arnella comes out with Edna who is calm and dressed in tan pants, white sweater and a floral blouse. Mr. Feldman, Arnella, Chevelle and Justine walk to a private part of the Pavilion, absorbed in conversation.

Later in the day, Justine relates the trouble of dressing certain residents:

> I have told Louis, "What works for you might not work for me, you see? We have to do what is best for us and make sure that they get the proper care." It's even gotten to the point when they (family members) go up to the office to report us for the way we handle her. It's because it takes all three of us to dress Edna because one is witnessing that the others are not abusing her. She screams and hollers like somebody is hurting her. She will kick, scratch and bite. Her husband didn't like the fact that there were three of us.

In the public space of the Pavilion, a few early-risers are ambling along the corridor. A buzz of conversation fills the air. CNA Glenda heads for the linen cart to pick up sheets when resident Miss Ava Reynolds screams, "Leave my damned stuff alone. Leave my cart alone. That's mine. The man told me to do that. That's my job." Miss Ava (also known as Aunt Ava) is an 81-year-old African American who has been on the Pavilion for three years. Fiery and stubborn, Miss Ava Reynolds is a favorite of CNA Justine. Aunt Ava comes from a background of hardship. At a young age, she put her husband in the grave and her three children through school. Always a domestic worker, she enjoys smoking a cigarette every now and then when she goes to the canteen with Justine.

Glenda walks over to Ava, and says, "This is not your job, you *used to* work." Glenda's tone of voice is firm but gentle at first. "You're not working any more. This is my job now. You're retired. You rest now, Miss Ava." "You're a damned liar," Ava shouts. "You better leave my stuff alone." Ava comes over, wraps her hands around the cart handle and pushes. Glenda repeats, "Go have a seat now, Ava. This is NOT your cart." As Aunt Ava's voice grows louder, so does Glenda's. The two hit a perfect match of octaves when Miss Ava backs off, pouts, and calls out to another CNA, "Sister, sister, come and get this woman." Before Glenda can respond, Miss Ava plops in the nearest chair and looks around the room in seeming defeat. "If she comes and wants to take it from me, then I have to get the tone she has and kind of holler back," Glenda tells me. "You have to get on that level with her. The same level that she gets with you. You have to be firm." "Does it work," I ask. "Yea, it really works. Then she'll calm down and want someone to help her." Different CNAs have different approaches to Aunt Ava under different circumstances. Glenda's approach may not work and may call for a different interaction situated in understanding and embedded in figuring out "where Miss Ava is coming from," one of Justine's skills.

Before breakfast I leave the sitting area and walk toward the restroom but am distracted by loud talk coming from resident "Boots" Jarrett's room.[2] The door is ajar[3] and I hesitate, not wanting to intrude into the scene. Both Marita and Boots are sitting on the bed with their backs to me. Boots, still in her nightgown, is shouting, "Goddam it, go to hell. No!" Marita is responding to her but I cannot make out what she is saying. Her voice is very soft as she takes Boots' hand in hers but Boots jerks it away. Marita turns and walks over to the sink where she picks up a container half-filled with warm water and a plastic bottle with a pink substance in it. She walks back to the bed and eases in beside Boots who is looking out the window. She empties a bit of the pink substance into the water and swishes it around with a washcloth. After ringing some of the water out of the cloth, Marita places it on Boot's shoulder. "Get away," Boots utters in an angry tone, but Marita strokes her shoulder and moves across her back only stopping to refresh the cloth with warm water. Boots, whom the CNAs know to be hot-tempered, is stilled by Marita's touch as she continues to stroke her back up and down. After several minutes, Marita goes to the closet to get Boots' clothes for the day and I take my leave. Later in the day I ask Marita to tell me about her approach with Boots:

> When I went in there, I approached Boots and said "good morning." She was just angry. So I had some lotion that I put in her wash pan. See, I'm an old nurse's aide. I'm from the school way back when. I warmed the lotion up and put it in the water and by the time that I finished washing her up and put the lotion on her back and everything, it was nice. She changed from an

> angry person to a pleasant person, but it all depends on the approach in the morning. If that's how you wake them up in the morning. If you go in there and just don't say nothing. I wouldn't want that for myself. I wouldn't want that for any of the people that I know and love. You have to have tenderness for them. There is always a psychology of the person. You have to understand that the illness is dementia. I'm going to give an example. When you go into a room, you want to be greeted with a good morning. This is bed and body that I am talking about. The approach in the morning, the way you wake up in the morning, that's the way you're going to have your day. And I want the CNAs to be concerned about the introduction for that day to the patient. "Good morning. How are you doing?" Just have some kind of pleasant conversation, a good greeting. And the way you do that, psychologically, you're getting them ready for whatever it is they're going to do when they walk out that door. And I know this for a fact.[4]

"Stop Joan—NOW! She's on the move again," screams Arnella. Resident Joan Ryder is on one of her morning rants, going from room to room "trashing" (unmaking) freshly made beds. This morning the staff surveillance of Joan's whereabouts lapsed long enough for her to hit three rooms. Chevelle runs to Miss Ava Reynolds' room, stops Joan in mid-trashing, takes her by the arm to the big blue sofa in the family room, and sits beside her. I cannot hear the conversation because Marge Jacobs is in fine form at this hour, her thunderous chant booming across the room, "One, two, THREE, Out goes SHE into the DEEP BLUE SEA, Seven eleven, BASEBALL SEVEN ELEVEN, Deep blue seeeeaaa …" Then, as quickly as Marge's mantra envelops us, she falls silent.

On the far side of the Pavilion the morning ceremonial of staff greeting residents as they come to breakfast is underway. There is a sublime quality to the quietude. The day seems, in resident Paulina Creed's words, "to have promise." A few of the residents, Boris Randolph, Carrie Mae Gordon, Roy Mitchell and Edna Feldman have come to the tables. Edna Feldman looks up and smiles. We talk about the breakfast foods and she tells me she likes cold cereal and fruit. Each resident is being greeted and welcomed to another day by the staff. Chevelle and Carma Lee bring Ruby into the breakfast table. She is skin and bones. The short sleeves of her safari smock create hollow dark circles out of which her fragile arms extend. She is recovering from a hip fracture. She walks as though each step represents an act of sheer will and triumph over falling. Ruby looks more frail than usual this morning. Gently, CNAs help her into the chair as she sinks in and almost disappears in its contours. Justine greets her with, "Hi Ruby, you want a cup of coffee?" Something prompts Grace to ask Ruby where her home is. Ruby cannot make out what Grace is asking her and says, "What?" followed by "oh, forget it, shut up." CNA Justine, who has been watching the exchange, picks up the threads of the question and says, "Ruby, she just wants to know where your home was." Ruby will get angry from time to time with other residents, but not with the staff.

Justine continues to arrange the utensils at the residents' places, her body turning rhythmically inward toward the residents as she moves around the table.

Justine looks up as she pours orange juice, and casts her eyes toward Isabelle inching down the corridor. "Girl, is that Isabelle comin' in?" It is as though there is an event each time a resident comes toward the table. Justine and the other CNAs are the welcoming committee. Justine's tone is one of recognition, affirming the adult person who is joining them. CNA Arnella, who is keeping things going at the table, takes the cue from Justine, catches Isabelle's eyes, clasps her hand, and walks them to the table. Arnella lowers Isabelle inch by inch into a seat at the table's end. Relief is written all over Arnella's face because the interactive experience with Isabelle doesn't always work. Then, there's "hell to pay" according to CNA Chevelle. Isabelle can be a biter and a fighter. Removing the brush from her pocket, Arnella grooms Isabelle's hair. She gives two substantial strokes to straighten out the neck-length silver mane. Isabelle is a handsome woman with a stately bearing. After Arnella has brushed her hair and after Isabelle has ceased the rhythm of leaning into each and every stroke, she takes Isabelle's hand in hers, caresses it, and lingers for a moment.[5]

"Well look who's coming—Aunt Ava," Justine calls, "you're up early this morning." An air of expectancy arises as each resident is brought in by the staff. Charge Nurse Marita Martin joins the group commenting she will feed Bertha Waker this morning. "I made the mistake of not feeding her yesterday and she was mad at me all afternoon," Marita says and glances at Bertha with a respectful twinkle in her eye. Yet another practice is about to take place in the way Marita eases into the seat next to Bertha, looks into her eyes and peers at Bertha for a moment to establish her presence. Marita opens the white can of Ensure supplement and stirs it as she continues to hold Bertha's gaze. She primly takes the spoon out of the folded napkin and unwraps it. With a certain focused artistry, she dips the spoon into the cereal with crisp care and lifts it to Bertha's face, catching any remains that land on her lips. Timing, patience, and establishing quiet are crucial.

Resident Sally Golden breezes by and CNA Carma calls to her, "How are ya doin'?" "Tryin' to find my home," Sally replies. She goes into Boris Randolph's room and closes the door behind her. Resident Max Campbell and Harriet French are methodically walking in and out of resident rooms. Max assumes his characteristic pose as he peers into the room first, looks either way, and enters as if looking for something. When questioned by a CNA, he says he is looking for his "lost room." On the opposite side of the Pavilion Bernice and Grace are making their turns around the corridor that encompasses the sitting area. The CNAs are very clear about the meaning they attach to the residents' movement and pacing throughout the Pavilion. They interpret such walking as the natural outcome of being housed in a confined space, that is, "feeling trapped" (from my discussions with the staff I can conclude their meaning would incorporate being trapped in psychic space as well).

Without warning, the fire alarm explodes in the room. Marita screams, "Anne, stop him, he's against the fire door trying to leave." I turn my head to see that respite care resident, Abe Levy, with his strong body and even stronger will, has managed to jar the door. "Talk to him, talk to him," Marita screams. I jump up and rush to the door to stop Mr. Levy though not without some struggle and a reference to his wife with whom I share a first name. "Anne will be here to pick you up very soon," I say, going eye to eye with him as he waves his arms above his head to escape my grasp. Much to my relief, Arnella and Glenda come to my rescue. They each lock their arms around Abe's arms, one on the right and one on the left, and walk him to the sitting room. All the time they murmur to him that his wife is coming to take him home. Mr. Levy had attempted to leave previously, but that time the results were very different. Marita Martin's arm was broken. Her family wanted her to sue but she refused. Now, she would talk to Abe and try persuasion. This incident gives me a chance to feel one short occasion of the physical and psychological demands Marita Martin and her team of CNAs confront. Afterward, I melt into a chair in the sitting room and don't budge for a long time.[6]

Henrietta Stein comes over and says "Hi" and wants to know how I am. Looking at the clock she asks, "When will we have lunch?" CNA Diane tells her about 12:30. The preparation of residents for lunch at the Pavilion commences around 11:30. CNA Glenda is going around to the aides and taking orders for burgers at McDonald's. The delivery of the food trays on time seldom happens. Henrietta Stein is getting very excited about whether she is going to get her food when she wants it and resorts to shouting, "BRING it down here. Come on and bring it down here," she yells at the top of her lungs. Her tone sounds as though she has willed it to be an octave higher as she barks her command to the CNAs. Carma Lee, who is rolling a resident into the dining area, looks over and calls to Henrietta, "Someone is hungry." With that, Henrietta gives her a hard as nails stare and heads for the family room out of sight. CNA Arnella interprets Hennie's yelling as "One of her plays for attention. She tries to control the CNAs."

Just at that moment, resident Roy Mitchell, who is sitting at the end of the long table, bursts into song with "I-I-I-I-I…'ve been workin' on the railroad" and there is a quick hush of residents and CNAs as they listen to Roy. He has a beautiful, full voice and is so robust in belting out the tune that his suspenders and bow tie are quivering. We're caught up in his energy and boldness. Myron, the maintenance man, calls, "Hi, Hennie. How are you?" "Fine when I see you," she replies. Now Roy has switched to "A-A-A-A-A…in't a gonna' rain no more, no more, ain't a gonna' rain no more …" Each word is crystal clear and ringing into the room. Resident Julia is tapping her feet and Grace is moving and singing.[7] In a few minutes, Henrietta gets serious again. "When are we eating?" "In about ten minutes," CNA Diane replies. "Clean off the tables … please," Henrietta requests. Turning toward me with a smile on her face, CNA Diane whispers, "I knew that was comin'." "It's after twelve o'clock," Henrietta replies. Now everybody gathers into singing again. "Take me out to the ball game …," Roy croons. CNA Carma Lee calls, "Lunchtime everybody."

From the family room come the plaintive sounds of Henrietta who is now half-sprawled across the sofa with one leg draped over the side of the cushion, her toe grazing the floor. She moans, "I am sick. I'm sick at my stomach." Her tongue hangs out, the back of her right hand rests on her brow, and her left hand clutches her abdomen as though writhing in pain, all reminiscent of a wild west drama in which one of the characters is not long for this world. CNA Arnella walks over to tend to Henrietta, a smart 94-year-old whom the staff assert is "not a true Alzheimer's." As I follow, Arnella whispers to me that this is " another one of Hennie's plays for attention."

At long last, there is the sound of trays being lifted from the food carts. Most residents are seated at the dining table. These are the sights and sounds of today's lunchtime scene:

> "I would certainly like to eat NOW," calls out Henrietta Stein who is already at the table … "Out goes she into the middle of the deep blue sea …" "Let's put this around your neck so you won't mess up your dress …" (things get quiet for a minute) … "Put this around you so you won't mess up your clothes, Martin." "Sit Harriet, where are you going? … "Come on it's almost lunchtime, yeh come on …" CNA Glenda goes over and fiddles with the piano, "Yes I'm just a prisoner of love" is coming from the stereo … Time on everyone's hands … "Sit down dear … You need to sit down …" "No, you're fine right where you are …" Marge shouts in the background, "1, 2, 3 Out goes she in the mid…dul … of …" A couple of aides are chuckling at a joke one of them is telling … Marge comes over to me and says, "I try to make a softball of this." "Did you do it," I ask. Marge replies, "This is one did one thing and one thing another. Out goes she in the middle of the deep blue sea …" CNA Carma Lee joins her, "1,2,3, out goes she." "Play us a song, Glenda …" "Marge, don't hit yourself like that …" CNA Glenda is at the piano … "You could play the 'Bugle Boy of Company "C"'" … "How many do they have in the middle of the deep blue sea? …" "I don't want to stay in this building all the time and I want to go to Cleveland," says resident Elnora as she strides by me … "We need some food over here … a tray please …" "Soon as they bring 'em over I will *get* you one, Hennie."

Boris Randolph, Carrie Mae and Paulina Creed talk among themselves even though understanding may be limited. Others with heads bowed await encouragement from the CNAs. Her manners very much in tact, Ruby Klein gets very angry at those who take food from another's plate as she sometimes accuses Hennie of doing. Other residents fixate on what is happening around them but also may help one another with finding the right utensil or finding a napkin. Those with the slowest movement, the hands curved from arthritis, the small inching of the finger and the hand hovering over the food, are unsure what to do, how to cut, but discover that pulling works. They bring the bite to their mouths and land it on the tongue all the while perhaps engrossed in some other place or time. The hats, the jewelry, bespeak the individuality and social class of residents.

"Something Violent"

When I return to the Pavilion after lunch on this mid-winter day, a sour smell hits me as I enter the open space of the dining and living areas. No residents greet me this afternoon. While some residents are in the bathrooms at this hour, Edna, Moselle and Henrietta are still at the dining table in the aftermath of lunch. Moselle is rubbing her fingers in the liquid food on the table with complete absorption, as though finger painting. Residents are fixed on parts of their bodies or on the objects before them. Martin Lovett sits in a pool of sunlight at the end of the table, shredding little pieces of paper onto the table top. I go over and touch his shoulder, calling his name. He does not stir. There is a heaviness in the air unlike other times when things feel lighter, brighter. I remember what CNA Diane Johnson said about different "atmospheres" on the Pavilion that seem to catch everyone, creating a world of contrasts. This resembles a "blue" afternoon as CNA Carma Lee puts it.

I look around for Marita Martin and the CNAs. Most of them are gathered in the nurses' alcove, which is very unusual at this time of day when toileting residents is the priority after lunch. There has been an accident, "something violent," Chevelle tells me.

> Mary was taking a short nap. When the substitute CNA went to get Mary up, she didn't want to be bothered. Mary lashed out at her and hit the girl hard in the eye and gave her a black eye.

This worker had been trained by the CNAs in skillful ways to approach Mary but this time it didn't work. "Earlier this morning, when we gave her a bath, she scratched and tried to bite me," Chevelle remarks. She then reveals the social and personal consequences in dialogue with me:

CHEVELLE: It's not easy to communicate. It looks easy, but it's not. You have to deal with so many of them and each one of them is different. But in another way they are all alike. Two of 'em spit a lot. Louisa, she fights you. Miss Ava, she will give you a good hit if you're not careful.

ANNE: Do you ever feel anger when this happens?

CHEVELLE: Yes, you have to deal with a lot dealing with the different levels of these people. You have to be watching, listening. Maybe when I get home it can take two hours to wind down. It's hard mentally.

For Chevelle, who has been hit by residents several times, the social consequence is internalizing her anger while she is on the Pavilion; the personal consequence is carrying the experience home where she can "wind down" on her own time. On one level this shows remarkable restraint, attitudes and practices that are collectively honored and enforced within the work group. But on another level, it highlights that things don't always go smoothly, that unpredictable things happen to staff, that violence, racist comments and other insults do happen. Marita tells me when she gets home, "It is two or three hours before I can take my 'suit' off."[8]

CNA Justine interrupts our conversation, "I just can't deal with it today. I'm going off. I've got to leave for a while. Maybe my sister will be in the canteen and we can talk a bit. Tell Marita I'm taking a break." Arnella, Chevelle and Carma Lee nod as Justine makes a beeline for the door and disappears from the Pavilion. Later in the day, Justine explained her urgent need to leave the Pavilion and give herself a "breather." She tells me about her self-reflection as she talks to herself in the canteen:

> When I get ready to go back, I say, "OK, I'm going to deal with this and I've got to handle it. Get on back there and deal with the problem." I think that's the way it is with all of us.

Justine gets headaches, Carma Lee can have a "blue" day, while Chevelle doesn't know "where my brain is sometimes." Evidence of stress and coping take different forms. Marita commented to me that "the girls have such control. Nobody (on the outside) has any idea how much."

I make my way over to the sitting area where "quiet time," a period initiated by LPN Marita when lights are lowered to calm residents after lunch, has just begun. Loud discussion is coming from across the room. Leona Phillips is standing in the middle of the room taking off her plaid dress and revealing her sheer nightgown underneath. Resident Ruby Klein is so disturbed by this that she tells Grace Bradford seated next to her to look at what is happening. They both eyeball Leona. "What's wrong with you? What king of person would take their clothes off? Are you crazy? What's wrong with you?" tiny Ruby screams. "Go to hell." Arnella goes over to Leona, takes her arm and walks her to her room.

The Pavilion grows quiet as I find a seat next to Henrietta Stein. This afternoon there is talk of birds in the courtyard as CNAs sit with the residents in the living room area. The lights are purposely low, the television silent, and the soft hum of workers' voices assume a complementary cadence to the residents' napping sounds. Drowsiness is everywhere. We are roused from our lethargy by the rhythmic sounds of:

> *Once upon a midnight dreary, while I pondered, weak and weary, Over many a quaint and curious volume of forgotten lore, While I nodded, nearly napping, suddenly there came a tapping, As of someone gently rapping, rapping at my chamber door. "'Tis some visitor" I muttered, "tapping at my chamber door; Only this, and nothing more."*

Heads turn. CNAs cease their activity. An insistent "Shhhh" is coming from those who are near resident Marge Jacobs as she dance-steps to the edge of the sitting room. We all become fixated on Marge as she moves to the family room's center. "Oh my," Marita Martin says, locking eyes with Arnella across the room. Marita whispers to the rest of us, "She did all the stanzas of the poem a while back and we couldn't believe it. But now …"

> *Deep into the darkness peering, long I stood there, wondering, fearing, doubting, dreaming dreams no mortals ever dared to dream before; But the silence was unbroken and the stillness gave no token, And the only word there spoken was the whispered word, Lenore? This I whispered, and an echo murmured back the word, "Lenore!" Merely this, and nothing more.*

Marge's voice rings with fervor, varying in intonation as the phrases spill from her lips. CNAs gather along the perimeter of the sitting room …

> *Open here I flung the shutter, when, with many a flirt and flutter, In there stepped a stately raven, of the saintly days of yore. .... perched above my chamber door, just above my chamber door, perched, and sat, and nothing more. .... Take thy beak from out my door. Quoth the raven, "Nevermore." Poe.*

Marge Jacobs pauses and then finishes her partial recitation of Edgar Allen Poe's *The Raven* with, "Out goes she into the deep blue sea, softball seven-eleven …" Silence fills the space. Marge looks up and around and all of a sudden spontaneous clapping breaks out as she dances toward the edge of the room. "Great job," CNA Arnella calls to Marge. "Thank you." Keeping perfect time and dancing in place, Marge moves into her normal pattern of speech that the CNAs call "rhyming." "Softball seven eleven. Out goes she into the deep blue sea. One, two, three, out goes she, seven eleven, seven eleven." With that, she step-skips down the corridor.

Liveliness in residents asserts itself in many other ways as well. Harriet French may kiss you one minute, slap you the next and mesmerize you as she plays the piano encouraged by the presence of the CNA Glenda who nestles beside her on the bench. Harriet can bathe the Pavilion in beautiful music amidst the rattling of trays and "busyness" of residents as they walk or talk. As CNA Chevelle says, "Some of 'em have those moments when it's almost like they don't have dementia. It's amazing. They make so much sense."

The following interchange with 94-year-old Henrietta Stein is even beyond making "so much sense" and thrills one with the nuance and humor of her comeback. One day on the Pavilion she was asking me my "maiden name" and the following took place:

> Kemp. K-E-M-P. There were some people who owned a bank at 13th and Saluta Street. That great big bank. And their name was Kemper. Lot of money. The First National Bank. Are you related to those people?

No, unfortunately not. (we both chuckle) I wish I were.

Yeah, I wish you were *effectively* related.

Yeah, If I were effectively related I might be able to get your million dollars for you.

Yeah (big laugh).

Day after day I witnessed an intricate entanglement of confusion and crystal clarity among the residents. Earlier today just after breakfast, resident Edna Feldman comes forth with a burst of clarity as CNAs Arnella, Chevelle and I are sitting alongside her in the dining area. Edna is weak and disoriented. She is playing with her bib, which is covered from end to end with fragments of food and stains along with her hands and fingernails. Her eyes, however, are bright when she smiles. She fiddles with the bottom of the bib, folding it over and over as though wanting to attach it to the table apron. All of a sudden, she looks up and says:

EDNA: You know, I never drove a car.

ARNELLA: I didn't know that.

ANNE: Do you miss driving a car?

EDNA: (With a split-second turn of her head, she looks at me dead on) I never drove. How would I know? Arnella and Chevelle are beaming as they look at me.

ANNE: You're right. How would you know if you never had the experience (all the while smiling at my lapse and her crystal clear and incisive comeback).

As the day shift ends, CNAs are busy doing their charting. Marita and Justine stay beyond the 3:00 pm official end of their shift several times a week and this is one of those days.

Life on the Pavilion is a study in contrasts, contradictions and unpredictability. In the midst of unintelligibility, disorientation, and profound confusion, remarkable intellectual vitality and creativity can arise from residents. I witnessed this emergent vitality in the residents often during my time there. At the same time, I observed sudden outbursts of anger and sometimes physicality. Staff face an ongoing difficulty in such a fluid environment. Allowance of time with each resident is a hallmark of the CNAs care work as opposed to speed and efficiency, the driving force of routinized, highly regulated care.[9] CNAs try to employ a rhythm in their care work, *a way of being*, as they strive to "make time" instead of being "made by time."

Herein lies a dilemma. On the one hand, staff members favor quiet for purposes of opening lines of communication with residents. On the other hand, they want to allow as much freedom as possible to "let the residents be" which accommodates, if not invites, speaking, singing, and yelling on the Pavilion. Part of the Starrmount CNAs' ongoing struggle is maintaining the delicate balance between quiet and clamor in an environment teeming with unpredictable resident action. Marita instituted a quiet time in the afternoon after lunch when lights are turned very low so silence can take root for twenty minutes, an eternity for some of the residents. She believes that intentional quiet can calm the residents even with Marge Jacobs rhyming and moving along the corridor. Although one cannot know for sure, Marita may be predicating her idea on the possibility that residents have become habituated to Marge's chant, a droning sound in its regularity, something akin to a loud air conditioner. Marge's chant, however, can provoke others when she is face-to-face with any one.

Another way quiet and taking time are established is by going to a center atrium in the Pavilion away from the family room when Marita senses that a resident is seeking a meeting with her. From time to time, Boris Randolph and his lady friend, Carrie Mae, meet with Marita to talk about taxes and having money for Carrie Mae to buy rouge when she needs it. Boris Randolph's desire to have such a meeting can become urgent, his demands persistent and his temper red hot. LPN Marita takes these occasions seriously because she and the CNAs know that "When you jump into their world with them it calms them down. We've been doing it all along." In fact, the care workers at Starrmount were continually constructing individualized strategies to understand and communicate with each resident and to create rhythm and routine amid a fluid setting.

In his classic ethnography of a nursing home, *Making Gray Gold: Narratives of Nursing Home Care*, Timothy Diamond provides a rich analysis of the lives of residents and the demanding work of nursing assistants. Frontline workers in Diamond's study labor under routinized, bureaucratic conditions in contrast to Starrmount CNAs who have the relative autonomy to construct and implement what they refer to as "different care."[10] In his study, Diamond identified what he called "mother's wit," a term used by one of his teachers in the school he attended to become a nursing assistant. Speaking to the challenges of being a nursing assistant, his teacher stressed, "What this work is going to take, is a lot of mother's wit. Use it and you'll stay out of trouble." Diamond remarks, "Her phrase stayed with me all the time I was working in the homes." He interprets this wit as distinctly "maternal feeling and skills."

In contrast, Marita Martin and the Starrmount CNAs did not characterize their work as maternal or gender-specific but referred to their skills and knowledge as a "different" kind of care. Diamond uses mother's wit as the base from which to call for a "vocabulary of care" in future research. *Women of Color in a World Apart* responds to Diamond's call through the demonstration and explication in detail of a "language of care" developed by Starrmount CNAs.

Notes

1 Jaber Gubrium coined the phrase, "bed and body" work to describe the multiple tasks and hands-on care that nurse's aides perform for patients in the nursing home in *Living and Dying at Murray Manor* (New York: St. Martin's Press, 1975: 59).

2 Verna Morris, known as Boots, was an independent, strong woman who raised her children to be the same. Her daughter, Toni, a successful businesswoman who travels, is close to the CNAs and comes often to the Pavilion when she is in town. She told me that she can "relax" when she is there, "let my hair down" so to speak. She likes to talk to the residents and enjoy herself.

3 I did not go into residents' rooms unless invited by the resident or staff. When the door was slightly ajar, I made a decision to observe or turn my eyes away depending on what is going on in the room and how intimate it is. I relied on reports from CNAs on activities within the resident's room. Since residents are outside of their rooms for the greater part of the day, this was not a liability. On one occasion, the privacy of a resident, Martin Lovett, was exposed because Arnella had hurried him from the main sitting area due to bowel incontinence and did not have time to close the door.

4 For Marita, the psychological is embedded in bed and body work with the resident, not a separate sphere. Marita's skill is influenced by her cultural background, growing up in a Mexican-American family. She had a strict father who awakened her in the morning with only a curt, "Get up," devoid of warmth. She mentioned that she hated that approach which could sour her own mood for the rest of the day.

5 Considerable skill goes into understanding when, for how long, and in what context Arnella and the other CNAs can touch Isabelle without her becoming highly agitated and refusing to eat. Isabelle is very stiff this morning and it takes forever for Arnella to get her to the table as they move inch by inch, Isabelle shuffling and trying to wriggle her arm from her companion's grasp. CNAs must execute the tiniest movements with interminable patience to establish an emotional and physical connection with Isabelle for each task during the day. The importance of Justine's individual recognition of Isabelle, saying her name out loud, and announcing her arrival in public (the group) cannot be underestimated as preparation for Arnella having the best possibility of completing the task of Isabelle's eating and grooming. The "breakfast ceremonial" carries important practical and symbolic meaning. Here is where the power of ritual replaces routinization, the sine qua non in institutional life. As opposed to a set of rules, standardized behavioral norms, and a strict schedule that never varies, the CNAs' approach serves to acknowledge individuality, to help establish membership in a group, and it marks the beginning of the day. The CNAs' approach privileges spontaneity, individual identity. It provides, also, an important control of behavior while not sacrificing one of the important tenets of the CNAs—responding to the emotional needs and well-being of the residents. The redundancy of the interactional ritual and its rhythmic tempo each day appear to have a calming influence on all. On the complexity of care work as combining both skills and feelings, see Emily Abel and Margaret Nelson, "Circles of Care: An Introductory Essay," in Emily Abel and Margaret Nelson (eds), *Circles of Care: Work and Identity in Women's Lives* (Albany, NY: State University of New York Press, 1990: 4–34), and Hilary Graham, "Caring: A Labor of Love," in Janet Finch and Dulcie Groves (eds), *A Labor of Love: Women, Work and Caring* (London: Routledge & Kegan Paul, 1983: 13–30). Also see emotion work in Jason Rodriquez, *Labors of Love: Nursing Homes and the Structures of Care Work* (New York: New York University Press, 2014: 115–137); As well, see Mignon Duffy, Amy Armenia and Clare Stacey (eds), *Caring on the Clock: The Complexities and Contradictions of Paid Care Work* (New Brunswick, NJ: Rutgers University Press, 2015).

6 Care work involves dimensions of power and control, even while these forces can be exercised humanely. While power may be present in all social practices it does not mean that all power is equal: there are different kinds of power, exercised in myriad ways.

The staff attempt to understand residents and "where they are" and direct their skills gleaned from ongoing relationships with the residents to a variety of different ends, including a form of personalized, individualized humane care as well as control. Some would argue that the use of coercion and restraint can require a lot of effort and is costly, leading CNAs to prefer tactics that try to convince the other to accept and voluntarily go along with control efforts. While Starrmount CNAs and Marita may agree in certain situations, such as the one with Abe Levy, the issue is more complicated for this group of women. They also *prefer* approaches that try to convince the resident to accept and go along with control not just because it is less costly and easier, but because it is consistent with their principles of care. A key part of the CNAs' skill involves knowing the nuances of just when and how to gain control and when to relinquish it.

7 The CNAs, Marita, and some residents will join in spontaneous bursts of collective exuberance, sometimes with fragments of word and melody, sometimes with clarity of lyrics. The sensual and social impact is akin to a collective high-spiritedness. The experience of a "rush of energy," even in day-to-day interactions, may kindle a solidarity among people, particularly when it can be sustained. The isolation imposed by dementia on the deepest level, which we cannot understand, may be lifted for residents, if only momentarily, by such an experience. There is no technique here, no set of rules to bring about "organized happiness," (I thank my colleague, Kassim Kone, for this phrase full of wit and wisdom) as if that were even possible. The singing comes out of the transitory ebullience of a kind of organic whole, which may have been fostered over time by the social relations on the Pavilion. This phenomenon is very similar to what Emile Durkheim calls "collective effervescence" in his classic book, *Elementary Forms of Religious Life*, ed. by Mark S. Cladis and translated from the French by Carol Cosman (New York: Oxford University Press, 2008 [1912]).

8 Shedding one's "suit" may be taking off protective armor after a contest of wills and emotions.

9 For an insightful study see Daniel Chambliss, *Beyond Caring: Hospitals, Nurses and the Social Organization of Ethics* (Chicago, IL: University of Chicago Press, 1996: 40), in which he focuses on the power of routinization. The uniformity of procedure and social control makes staff "normalize the abnormal," act in a businesslike manner to deal with what takes place in such a setting. Chambliss rightly emphasizes that routinization is much more than rules and a strict regulation of time, rather, it is a *way of being* that becomes "embodied in the nurse over time" and "globalizes to all life and care in the institution," to the detriment of care work. Also see Eviatar Zerubavel, *Patterns of Time in Hospital Life: A Sociological Perspective* (Chicago, IL: University of Chicago Press, 1979).

10 While both Diamond's nursing assistants and Starrmount CNAs experience intrusions into their work by regulatory agents, the degree to which this happens and its detrimental effects on the philosophy and execution of care work is much lessened at Starrmount. While different from my study in setting and purpose, Rodriquez's recent ethnography, *Labors of Love: Nursing Homes and the Structures of Care Work* (New York: New York University Press, 2014) argues that the bureaucratic nature of the nursing homes in his study allow for only scant autonomy for care workers; however, nursing assistants bring meaning to their work through forming emotional attachments to residents.

3

"GETTING INTO THE RESIDENT'S WORLD"

A central term in the language of care on the Pavilion was "getting into the resident's world." [1] I heard the staff use this phrase over and over to refer to how they were trying to decipher residents' own understandings and meanings of what was going on. While the entire interaction between staff and residents in this book exemplifies different ways that the staff attempted to get into the resident's world, this chapter addresses the phenomenon conceptually. Getting into the resident's world is a situationally grounded skill whereby staff orient to, and learn to use, residents' own understandings and meanings of the situation to better communicate. I found two overarching aims employed in this important skill: (a) meeting the emotional needs of residents and preserving dimensions of resident self and mind; and (b) discerning "where the resident is" in order to convince him or her to go along with certain staff concerns. As part of this process, care workers constructed what I term a "series of selves" to communicate with residents.

Boris Randolph, Carrie Mae Gorden and Ben Katz, a former business owner, gather in front of LPN Marita Martin's desk this Friday morning. The two men are intent on having a business meeting. They take full advantage of Marita's decision to remove the plexi-glass half of the alcove surround to confront her. Marita is absorbed in the daily routine of what she calls "endless, exhausting paperwork" about residents and the operation of the Pavilion. She greets the trio and tells them she can meet at 11:00 am in the large, private space between the ambulatory units, and the non-ambulatory third unit. Marita hopes to diffuse the group's anxiety about what they perceive is a money crisis by creating a business-like setting as she has done with Boris Randolph in their ongoing meetings. The group sits at a large, shiny table, not unlike a conference table. Ben lays out the problem:

BEN: You know, we're in need, all three of us.

MARITA: Well, what is it Ben?

BEN: You know kid, I hate to come to you but I know you'll trust me. I need $150. Could you spare it for the next two weeks? I'll give it back.

MARITA: Ben, you can have anything (writing his name and the amount).

BEN: Thanks a lot. (Ben sits there for a while and then slaps the table in front of Boris Randolph) OK, let her know what you want.

MARITA: Well, Mr. Randolph do you want me to draw money out of your savings account in your name?

BORIS: Oh, no, no, no. I just want an audit. I just want to know how much is in my account. (Turning to Carrie Mae and tapping her on the shoulder) Well, what about you, gal?

CARRIE: Could I have fifty dollars? I have to go to CATS (a local novelty store) and get some rouge.

BORIS: Rouge! Fifty dollars? (Mr. Randolph is getting loud and appears exasperated)

MARITA: Well, let me see what I can do for you …

When Marita tells Ben he can have anything he wants, this is not a delusion. Both men have large financial accounts.[2]

After the meeting I head back to the family room to sit with residents who have just finished lunch. Miss Ava Reynolds is pacing back and forth in front of the nurses' empty alcove. She looks angry, and presses her hands into the pockets of her yellow housedress. CNA Glenda tells me Ava is "pouting" and refuses to go to lunch. The staff will "wait it out" and return to her a little later to convince her to try some lunch fare. Discovering entry into Miss Ava's world is a challenge to the staff. When Ava, an "all-nighter," refuses to go to bed Justine tries to "see where Miss Ava is coming from":

> I know one night I worked 7 pm to 11 am. When I got here they said, "Miss Ava, she'll be up until tomorrow" (up all night). I said, "Why?" They didn't know. I looked over and asked Ava. "Do you remember crossword puzzles?" Ava just sat there … "You want to work first?" She said, "No." "You hungry?" She said, "Yeh." "Want to go to the canteen," I said. I didn't know she smoked. I gave her a cigarette. We just sat there and talked … I said, "Oh can you rub my neck?" She got up and rubbed until I thought I would go to sleep. I said, "Let me rub your neck." I rubbed. She said she was getting tired. I took her back to her room. I said, "I want you to lie down for a little while." She said, "OK." She went out. She had been up for maybe two days. They said they just couldn't get her to go to bed. But they just *told* her, "You got to go to bed." I tried to see where she's coming from.

Justine engages Miss Ava as a person. She offers her choices of action that provide for the possibility of shared experience between the two. The mutual neck rubbing and taking turns are acts of significance that affect future relations with the resident. Justine and Ava share an experience in a "bare bones" way in the canteen over a cigarette, letting their hair down together.[3]

As Hennie Stein leaves the lunch table she begins to dance, swaying her body, twirling her arms, her hands making little circles in the air. CNA Chevelle looks up and says with a smile, "Henrietta, (raising the pitch of her voice) you feel like dancin' this afternoon, huh?" Henrietta nods in rhythm with her movements as she promenades to the sitting area. CNA Glenda Morgan walks around issuing a proclamation, "The restaurant is closed now. The restaurant is closed. Come on, come on everybody. It's time to go." Marita explains how important money becomes and how they have been able to use it as a strategy for getting residents to and from the dining area. "It's a big one," Marita emphasizes.

> I reassure them about payment. If you tell them that the bill is already paid, "Well, who's paid it?" "Well," I say, "you've already paid your bill." "No, I haven't I haven't got a receipt." I get them one even if I have to write it out right there—"PAID."

Residents leave the table one by one, surveying the area in front of them, pondering their next move. Henry Mackey asks, "Well, what are we supposed to do now?" What is there to do now? One answer may be singing that begins with Recreation Leader, Diane Allen. Roy belts out a song, "The Little Brown Church in the Vale." His voice soars, and staff in the nurse's station listen to his clear baritone while doing paperwork. Resident Samuel Gold is at attention with his cane resting upright against his leg, one hand on the cane, the other holding his cup in the air as though giving a toast. Irene and Ada, arms folded, are on the couch in animated conversation. Roy Mitchell continues to survey the group while he sings. He has a cherubic face and a mischievous gleam in his eyes, and appears to know a little bit more about what is going on than what he is able to say, a people watcher.

In the corridor, Carrie Mae and Samuel Gold are headed somewhere. CNA Glenda asks them where they are going and they answer that they will be gone an hour. "Oh, you're going to be gone all that long?" They nod. "Well, ok, enjoy the time." The two of them continue to amble down the corridor. Glenda makes deft changes in intonation, word emphasis, and the use of an interrogatory sentence—"Oh, you're going to be gone *all that* long" which conveys a kind of affirmation of Sam and Carrie's reality. Using the pair's understandings of the length of their leave-taking, Glenda conveys acceptance and wishes them well. In other words, Glenda affirms a mutual understanding and even though she "had no idea" it would be that long, it's quite alright. It's never in question whether this is really happening, only a surprise at the length of time of "being gone" which further reinforces the "realness" of the experience for Carrie and Sam. Implicit in CNA Glenda's response to the pair is the crucial difference between *imparting support* and *issuing permission* to Carrie and Sam to exercise their "little freedoms," as Chevelle says, to move and "be gone" within the space of the Pavilion. Glenda participates in what I call "destinations of the mind" as well as protects the agency and personhood of both.[4]

CNA Justine speaks of achieving a deep empathy with the residents when she says,

> They're back forty or fifty years in their mind. Because everybody's mother and father is living. Everybody's always going to see Mom and Dad. Back to their hometown. They go back to the farm. So we have to get in with them. We have to go into their world with them. Whatever they're going through. We have to get in there and we go through that with them.[5]

Language describing entrance into the world of the resident has an intensity to it, connoting a sharing of attitudes. Words and phrases such as "jumpin' or climbing" into their world, or "going right in there with them," summon images of being in the midst of wherever the resident may be, in time and in action. These phrases suggest boundaries, an inside and an outside, and getting over an invisible barrier into another province of meaning. Staff do not hesitate at the periphery of this world as LPN Marita Martin reveals,

> What we're practicing now, it's been pointed out that it's a language. I understand him and he understands me. You just don't come by it in a day. It's more involved now. It's more intense. We're in this, I even want to say dementia. We can't talk any other way, like I'm talking to you. So we have to use what we have.

Sometimes, the intention for getting into the resident's world may be suspect as is evident in CNA Glenda's approach to Boris Randolph. In a desire to uncover racial prejudice and assess character, Glenda relates how she "tested" Mr. Randolph:

> Before I started to work here, someone told me Mr. Randolph was prejudiced and that he used to work in a bank. I asked him, "Mr. Randolph, I came to apply for a loan." He says, "Well you will have to fill out this application. I will not guarantee you will get it." I said, "Why? Is it because I'm Black?" "No, no. That's not the reason. That's not the reason. But that has happened in some cases," he told me. I wanted to see by my being Black, would he give me a loan, what his reaction would be.

This interaction could be interpreted as "setting up" Mr. Randolph, with Glenda using her power of intelligibility and his cognitive impairment so as to discover a "truth" and confront him. The exchange illustrates the ever-present temptation for the staff to take advantage of easy access to residents afforded by the absence of social and occupational barriers, particularly when it involves something as emotionally charged as potential racism. When I asked her why she did what she did, Glenda said it was because she wanted to get Boris Randolph's reaction. She did not seem to sense an ethical lapse in her behavior but appeared comfortable in her strategy. One may also understand this as Glenda Morgan's means of investigation, preparing herself to work with a majority of White residents.

The Series of Selves

Today is Valentine's Day and the Pavilion is decorated with pink and red hearts everywhere. Resident Carrie Mae lingers at the dining table after others have left and is in conversation with CNA Glenda. She gives Glenda a little pat on what she calls her "rear end," kidding Glenda about getting it out of the way when she leans in to gather up the trays. Glenda looks around good-naturedly, feigning a little gruffness and says, "What are you doing with *that* back there?" They laugh and kid about Glenda's substantial hips, as resident Verna chimes in giggling. There is a give and take between *persons*, as aide and resident touch each other's worlds during moments of shared humor.

From the staff's perspective, residents are persons with unique histories and identities. Thus, complete loss of self is neither *inevitable* nor *absolute* for residents during the course of their stay. Care staff work to maintain meaningful selves through a variety of strategies including multiplicity or "series of selves." [6,7]

The Storied Self`

As "quiet time" begins, Resident Fay Morgan is eager to get CNA Diane's attention. Fay was a grade school teacher who has twin sons. Fay appears worried:

FAY: Won't you come over and sit? I'm looking for Paul. I knew where he was but I can't find him now.

DIANE: Let me pull a chair over. I'm afraid I have forgotten who Paul is.

FAY: My husband. He's around here somewhere and I'm sure he would get you a chair.

DIANE: What does he look like?

FAY: A very good husband (laughs)

DIANE: I thought you were going to say a very good-*looking* husband.

FAY: Well, he *is* pretty good looking. I've always thought he was and I still do. Last night my boys were there and there were other boys who sure enough were in school and came over and talked to them. Well it's going to be an improvement and I hope he is going to get more out of school.

DIANE: I do too.

FAY: You can't take it like a dose of pills (laughs). You have to take it by the meaning you're getting and the cooperation of the family. And the families are pretty good in most cases. And their children are just that much better. Because the good parents are the ones that help a great deal. But things will come up in the family and there will be some extra traveling that they didn't know about. And one of the older parents had to go and had a bad case of sickness and she had to make arrangements and there were two or three things of that kind that happened. But bless her heart that's just a blessing. Not that they got sick but that they had someone who loved them enough that they wanted to help 'em. Next time come and bring your children. Don't you have any? I thought you had one or two? We had twins and as they get older they are getting more interesting.

Diane witnesses the re-telling of a story. Climbing into the resident's world and evoking a "storied self," as with Diane and resident Fay, can serve as impetus for, and sustaining of, the relationship between staff and residents.

A storied occupational self can arise when Ruby Klein addresses Arnella as an employee in her family-owned furniture store:

ARNELLA: Did you get enough lunch, Ruby?

RUBY: Yes, honey. Yes, it was good. But you know I don't eat much. You know you're one of my better workers (half smiling), because I don't catch you sitting down on my time.

ARNELLA: Well, thank you very much. I really try hard.

RUBY: I know you do. And I'm gonna give you some time off.

Turning away from their conversation, I catch Ruby Klein's comment that they "have a lot of merchandise in their store ..." According to Arnella,

> Ruby is a woman with a big heart. She's spunky and she's bossy. When her first husband died, she just picked up and took over. She was a lady ahead of her time back then. She was always on the go, always a take-over type person. I think that's where she gets her feistiness. And she's just so tiny and she'll just stand up and tell somebody off and say, "Get over there and sit down!"

Arnella's ability to use the resident's own understandings to get into her world has an element of the culturally gendered roles of the 1940s and 1950s with possible assumptions about the position of Blacks in the social order. CNA Arnella realizes that the family department store of long ago is a source of present occupational identity for Ruby. She cautions, however, against being "anxious or agitated" because the residents will "pick up your behavior." Arnella acquiesces to a role that defines her as an unskilled worker "under" Ruby. In reality, Arnella is a paraprofessional, CNA and CMT, with several years of medical experience in contrast to an unskilled worker in a department store of the 1940s. Within this interaction she is constructed as demoted and plays it out with a white owner of the business. On one level this is a reminder of her "place" as gender and class roles are played out between them. On another level it is true also that this interchange may be experienced as an equalizing of control or reversal of control: Who is in charge and who is directing or guiding whom? On yet another level, the role is accepted by Arnella because of the relationship she has with Ruby. The staff like Ruby's gutsy attitude.

When a resident speaks about the past there is a blur between the storied self who is speaking *out* of the past and the storied self who is speaking about the past from the standpoint of the present. The staff prefer to learn about the storied self "for themselves" rather than rely on secondhand information from the family. The one exception to that involves learning about the resident's functional likes and dislikes such as what he or she enjoys for breakfast, his or her prior sleeping habits, and other practicalities.

Lights come on at the end of quiet time when tall, African American resident Verna (Boots) Jarret sashays past us on her way to the dining table. CNA Glenda and I stare at Verna, look at each other, and shake our heads. "She's got style," I say. Nodding, Glenda evokes the storied self as a point of connection between resident Boots and herself:

> Verna's personality says that at one time in her life she really had it goin' on. She loves to dance and the way she walks ... Before Verna came over here she was across the way over there in her own apartment. You could see Verna out there with those high heels on and with the long cigarette holder, you know, (swaying her body as she tells this). She was kinda struttin'. And she was kinda sayin' somethin' ... and she's still sayin' somethin' (we both laugh). But she's kinda slowed down a little bit and she'll let you know it too. She still likes to dance. Still likes to smoke, but she can't walk in the heels anymore.

In this vivid portrayal, CNA Glenda appreciates Verna Jarret's flair and style. Through a storied self of the recent past, Glenda makes a connection between *then* and *now* to perpetuate a picture of a sense of agency and pride in the resident as "still sayin' somethin', still struttin'."

Getting into the resident's world of the storied self can give the staff more respect for the resident as Diane relates:

> There was this man who was here who would hit you and then run off. There was nothing you could do to work with him. We went to his wife's

house. He had made some beautiful furniture. The headboard of the bed, beautiful carving and tables. I had much more respect for that man. I felt so sorry for what had happened to him.

The New Self

As I prepare to leave at 3:00 pm, Marita Martin whisks by saying that she needs to tell me something that occurred since I was last in the Pavilion. "You know what, you can join us if you like," she says. Marita and Mary Louise are heading back to the middle sitting room to cut and style Mary Louise's hair, a potentially explosive situation because Mary does not want anyone touching her head. A hairdresser comes to the quiet sitting room and Marita sits with Mary Louise as she is having her hair cut. The space becomes a beauty salon. The physical environment is ample distance from the action in the family room. Potential eruptions from Marge's rhyming, Roy's singing and resident fighting are avoided. Mary Louise can be hot-tempered, so timing and approach must be precise, honed over time through Marita's relationship with Mary Louise and her husband.

Marita sits in a chair facing Mary, their knees slightly touching. The beautician snips Mary Louise's hair with a gentle touch. Marita bends over, her body extends toward Mary Louise, eyes concentrated on her, what Marita calls "letting her eyes be the windows to the resident." Mary Louise manages to get out "Thaaannnk Youuuu." Marita says, "Well, you're welcome." Mary Louise rarely speaks and her thank you takes great effort. Marita's body position in the chair is near enough to reach across the private space of each, but a secure distance so as not to frighten Mary. Several minutes pass before Marita touches Mary Louise. She establishes "just the right amount of eye contact" until she perceives relaxation in Mary's brow and a lessening of the tightness around her lips.

Marita clasps Mary Louise's hands. The blending of beings is impressive as is the serenity. Mary Louise is still and Marita's hands are the conduit for communication. It seems as though a balm passes through these hands. Presence. Marita's stroking is rhythmical as she glides up and down from wrist to upper arm, to shoulder and back with varying degrees of grip. She covers Mary Louise's hands with her own to rest a moment in one unbroken motion of touch. I catch a flicker of radiance in Mary's eyes and then it vanishes. In these few moments mixed with urgency (to keep Mary L. from lashing out) there is a message of acceptance. Yet, the knowing bond must be established over and over again as many times as needed. All fretting is silenced and the functional process and beautifying can take place.

MARITA: You see, it wasn't so hard was it Mary? It wasn't that difficult.
HAIRDRESSER: With Marita's good help.
MARY LOUISE: Ummm (a peaceful look comes over her face).
MARITA: (laughing) It's makin' me sleepy. I was going to fall asleep on Mary's lap.

LPN Marita and the CNAs know how tricky these transitions can be for Mary Louise. They can set off a cascade of biting and scratching. Most of the time, if the approach fails because Mary has been antsy before the hair grooming, Marita stops and tries again at a later time. Today, however, time is of the essence as Marita stressed, "I must get the hair looking just right because the daughter is coming from out of town." Looking "just right" means looking as close to how the daughter, who seldom visits, remembers her Mother in earlier times, before dementia. "Some families expect the *IM*—possible," Marita laments.[8] In contrast to Marita's experience, Chevelle has been bitten and scratched while bathing Mary Louise in the whirlpool. "You can't just learn this overnight," Chevelle says. "Everything can be *so* unpredictable every single day." The whirlpool is a trapped environment for both CNA and resident and leaving Mary Louise alone is not an option.

Different types of relationships generate different types of sensibilities. Other channels (touch, smell, facial expression, eye contact) become more intense, more meaningful when normal speech and cognitive capacities fail. Therefore, "felt meaning," not formal symbolic agreement, becomes a powerful form of communication. Since symbolization and symbolic interaction cannot always be counted on between staff and residents, meaning-making and sharing is largely felt meaning, rather than formal symbolic agreement, a "sympathetic identification." These levels of communication may not be readily discernable to the observer but may be felt by the participants.

CNAs and Marita engage and respond to that part of the resident, the new self, who is in the Pavilion now, even in the midst of the shifting past and present. For Mary Louise, Martin Lovett and several others, the new self is extremely limited in verbal responsiveness. In contrast, for other residents, there is an immediacy to the new self that requires a response. CNA Carma Lee speaks of residents in the Pavilion as "being in a community looking for new friends, almost like they're starting all over again. They kinda find their own way and are comfortable in that." She captures the general feeling of the staff that there is another beginning here for the residents. What family members may see as an absent self, not the person they know, the CNAs see as a new self with characteristics that engage them in the here and now. As an emerging part of the resident, there are, what I call, *traits of being* that both amaze and dismay the families of the residents. These traits include what families say they have never seen their family member do, singing, dancing, being very gregarious and open with people. These traits also include what society would call deviant or aberrant behavior, and what the medical model would define as "signs" of the disease: Marge's rhyming, "One, two, three, out goes she into the deep blue sea, softball seven eleven," along with her accompanying little dance step, and resident Evelyn's responding to others with "Boy, oh boy, that's for sure, that's for sure … Boy, oh boy, oh boy …" Staff join in Marge's chanting and rhyming, a striking example of "sharing attitudes," incorporating these identity sounds into the woman they have come to know. As Justine says, "It's just Marge being herself." The CNAs' interpretation of Marge's chanting constructs and retains a past identity, incorporating it into the present narrative and new self. Marge's rhyming becomes a part of life on the Pavilion as CNA Carma Lee explains,

> She says "softball seven" all the time. That's just something she says every day. Some other people don't understand that. You understand that because that's what they do every day. It just becomes a part of them and it's not out of place. When they stop, that's when it's out of place.

In addition to being a sign of "normality" in a resident, such "traits of being" have another meaning of significance for the staff. They represent a new self who acts, engages, is appreciated and suffers. These traits are not shunned by the staff nor seen as "alien," neither are they glorified. Marge's chants can drive some staff "crazy" at times when they can't hear the other residents or themselves speak. Some families and "traditional nurses" as RN Pressley calls them, point to Marge's rhyming as "out of control and offensive." What can be appealing to some can be appalling to others.

The Imagined Self

The staff take pride in pointing out the former occupational identity of residents, whether it be homemaker as in the life of Ella Larson or speech-maker as in the life of Marge Jacobs. When there is sketchy information in the resident's biography, staff create a "must have been." "You can imagine who they used to be. Proud people like us," Marita declares. CNA Arnella uses the imagined self and the storied self of Marge Jacobs to reflect on her own life:
When I look at my residents I bet that, once, this

> particular person was a brilliant person … like Marge. I was told by her family that she was very intelligent. She had the talent of being a speaker. She could get everybody's attention and that talent is still there because she can get our attention here on the unit. I just sit back and think that could be me one day. I just try and enjoy my life.

Staff seek a way of making sense out of behavior/actions they observe in the residents. They construct an imagined self as an organizing point to help them figure out a current problem with the resident by imagining the way "she or he and the situation might/must have been" and to create a wholeness out of fragmentation. CNA Arnella is one of two staff members who point out the connection between Marge as public speaker then and now. Implicit in the staff's construction of the imagined self is a desire to keep a continuity between the past and present.

Creating an imagined self may also fulfill a need to find a surviving self to reference when staff are surrounded by shadowy self-images of the residents.[9]

Through imagining a past self, the staff can develop strategies to control behavioral problems and to solve a riddle. CNA Justine discusses her puzzlement over Mr. Randolph's style of dress and behavior:

> When he first came, he was always trying to leave. I just imagine that he is a businessman and he put his hat on before he went somewhere. And then another resident came in, Michael Reardon. The two of them seemed to get along pretty good and Reardon is a businessman too. His wife is a resident upstairs (in the larger nursing home). Michael didn't wear a suit or hat or tie. So Mr. Randolph started coming out with just a shirt and didn't have that hat.

CNA Chevelle tries to make sense of a resident's behavior that is disruptive and frustrating to other residents and herself at times:

> Rachel is so bossy. She'll be talking to you one minute and then she'll hit you like that. Mostly, I think of Rachel because she'll be trying to fix their (other residents') clothes on them or say, "Come on. You go over here and sit down." She'll be trying to tell them what to do. Rachel must have been a pretty bossy lady (in the past).

CNA Chevelle uses the imagined self to confirm certain traits. In this case, however, she does not attribute bossiness to the disease. She makes clear distinctions between the person acting and the disease acting. The imagined self is used as a tool to understand or account for behavior in the present. The pathos of getting into the world of resident Marge Jacobs after her fall takes its toll on the Starrmount staff.

"Our Sun: We Had A Shield Around Her"

> *Marge was, well, a highly educated woman. Fluent speaker, brilliant. Sometimes you can tell. She loves to talk. Talk all the time.*
>
> *CNA Carma Lee*

Today, as I sit with residents in the family room, I'm taken by surprise as Henrietta Stein, all tidied up in full clothing, replete with signature head scarf, leans over my shoulder and says, "It's hell getting one of their baths." With that, Ruby Klein, who is sitting next to me, raises her head and scowls at Henrietta who retorts, "I'm not talking to you." Across the room, Roy Mitchell relaxes in the rocker and surveys the group with his bemused smile. At that moment we are all jolted by loud sounds coming from Marge Jacobs' room. Have things taken a turn for the worse two days after Marge fell and cracked her pelvis?

I rush to her room and pause at the door. The aides encircle her bed as Marge, in great pain, thrashes from side to side on the bed. Her body is black and blue from the fall and gaunt from not eating. It's hard to imagine how this frail body and person can have so much will and raw strength. The CNAs are trying to get her to take some liquid nutrients:

AIDE: Close your mouth ...
MARGE: (screaming) One, two, three, out goes she ...
AIDE: Open your mouth and eat this ...

Marge screams as the CNAs lean over her to offer the best comfort they can. Tension abounds, as if something will explode. "Eat, eat, we want you to have it," begs Arnella. "You need this. You need this, Marge." Word comes from LPN Marita that the doctor wants her "restrained better." Marita and her staff look at each other. What does he mean? Marita, who is stroking Marge's arm moves away from the bed and comes to stand by me:

ANNE: What are you doing now?

MARITA: Comfort. Comfort measures. We go in there and try to give tactile and verbal stimulation. Everybody goes in once in a while and sits with her. "Marita, I'm going to be in here, today," they will say. Since it's not a bath day, everybody's going in there more than usual. The people around the other departments come and they hear her and they wonder where she is. There's been a couple of comments made that we're not doing the right thing. But that's not up to us. That's the family. But I don't have to explain to anybody what we're doing down here.

ANNE: Would you have expected her to stay here?

MARITA: Yeah. The daughter and her husband, they latched onto whatever care we were giving her because they said if we take her over to the hospital there's no sense in us even remotely thinking that we're going to be able to visit with her every day because they have a business to run. They say that they know that when she's here she's going to be cared for.

Marita tells me that she and the CNAs have decided, for the time being, to resist the physician's restraining order. One of them will always be with her and satisfy the need to check her every hour.

Marge Jacobs is one of the favorites in the Alzheimer's Pavilion. From her first day she enlivened the Pavilion and became "our sun," according to LPN Marita Martin. Her condition improved after she was brought from a geriatric care home, as Justine likes to recount,

> They had put her in a room, tied her up, and gave her all that medication. Then she came over here with us. She stopped wearing diapers. They took her off all medication. She became the life of the party. She was a public

speaker. She's still a public speaker. That counting got mighty slow but she's still counting. We were all, ah, crazy about her. You know, she was sayin' something too.

Marita Martin takes my arm and moves me toward the door as though wanting to have some privacy to talk:

MARITA: We've all had a rough week because of Marge. We're worried and don't know what to do. We're *so* concerned.

ANNE: What's her condition now?

MARITA: I think that she's getting ready to leave us. I really do. I really believe that. The family has been extremely gracious with us. In talking with them, they don't want her to be plugged up to anything.

ANNE: And what would that be?

MARITA: They don't want her to have a tube to feed her. This isn't the quality of life that she would want. We all got together, the family, the daughter, the son-in-law and myself, and Ms. Pressley. We discussed the quality and dignity that she deserves. They decided that they do not want hospitalization. They want us to take care of her here and do what we can.

ANNE: What would be the difference if you took her to the hospital?

MARITA: She would be bodily restrained. Four-point restrained. They would have to have IVs which means they would have to put the board on her, on both arms so she wouldn't move. That just doesn't make any sense. At least here she would have the emotional support from everybody. You can feel when somebody is warm to you. The staff is thinking that we're going to care for her here the best that we can and attempt to give her what she needs. She's refusing food. She's refusing water. But, I've seen this before. Just leave me alone. Don't bother with me. Let me die with other people. So, I try to do what I can but it doesn't seem to be enough. Ms. Pressley called me yesterday and told me maybe this is overlapping with my mom's death. She told me I was doing all I can. She said she sees that I am frantic. I said I am frantic because I don't have an answer. I don't have control. I can't do anything. The girls look at me like "What now. What do you want us to do now?"

Time after time, with great care, each aide pulls the coverlet over Marge's exposed body when she knocks it off. Carma Lee has told me how important modesty is to Marge.

AIDE: Marge, please. Stop it, you're makin' a mess.

MARGE: In the middle of the deep blue sea … out goes she … 1, 2, 3, out goes she … in thu mid-dul of thu deep blue sea …

AIDE: (as she dispenses medication) Marge, you have got to have this. Now, stop it, come now, open your mouth.

Marge is desperate and jerks her head from side to side. Finally, she grasps the words to say it … "please take it away." Eating, a shared delight between Marge and Justine, becomes a skirmish. Justine recalls,

> I really liked the way she loved to eat. I'd say, "let's have something different." At first, she could hold a real good conversation. I took her to the canteen. Let her pick out whatever she wanted. We may eat in there or come back to the unit. She loved bananas. The way she loved to eat. The way she could just sit down and really make you laugh. She was somethin' else.

The CNAs face a dilemma of no small proportions over the physician's order to "force feed" Marge. They find themselves in a tug of war over honoring the rights of the resident, their complicated emotions, and the medical demands. They want to *save* Marge, have her "be like she was."

The bulk of bodies in the room, the physical strength, and gentle touch that must be summoned to meet and match that tiny wasting body are palpable. The CNAs lift, turn, and try to caress Marge as her arms flay against them.

> CNA: You drink it and we'll be through. That's my baby, that's my baby, yes … (as Marge takes a little liquid).

The tension, having mounted in voice and body, dissipates in relief. As witness to this distressing scene, holding my breath with alarm, the relief that the worst seems to have passed is palpable. I let out the air trapped in my lungs, turn and walk out of the room. Marge's body, nude from the waist down, makes me feel a deep intrusion into her privacy and wholeness. A few feet away is the world of talk and television in the resident sitting area. We leap over a chasm from gripping reality to the world of socially constructed niceties when a family member calls to resident Alice Hogan, "Alice, Alice, don't do that. Take your hands out of your pants."

At last, I hear Arnella say to Marge, "Now you go to sleep … We're going to give you some water and get you to sleep. You're going to bed, to sleep. You're going to feel better … now … now …" There is a mesmerizing quality in Arnella's tone as she gathers Marge into a gentle holding place. I seek out Marita to resume our conversation.

> ANNE: How do you sense the CNAs' concern?
>
> MARITA: They're being vocal. They're being very disgruntled by what's happened. They were standing around her bed the other day and just looking at her. All the staff. We were all standing around her and this brought to mind my mother and I told them, "She's not dead. She is not dead, girls." They kind of looked at me and everybody says, "Yea, you're right, she's not." Well then I told them we have to make her comfortable

and make it as livable for her condition as we can. So Justine comments, "It's difficult to keep a good woman down." So they felt better and kind of chuckled. I said, "Just think of all the things that she's done. How she's brought joy to our lives, and I'm sure that we've brought joy and pleasure to her life. So, that's our biggy right now. Let's just get her through this, whatever it is. Be it if she's going to get back up again and leave us."

ANNE: What are you giving her?

MARITA: What I'm doing now is that I'm not giving her anything during the day, any pain medication other than Tylenol. Probably around 2:00 if she just gets extremely rowdy, I'll give her Demerol. She's been so zonked out that we haven't been able to feed her or get her to drink. That's why I'm doing this because she needs some kind of nourishment. What I can't understand, one minute she's up and rambling around and she knows that she's hungry and she knows that she's thirsty and knows that she has to go to the bathroom. And then the next minute it's all gone. She doesn't know if she's hungry, if she's thirsty. She doesn't know that she has the urge to urinate. And this happened in one day.

ANNE: From the fall you're talking about?

MARITA: Yes. Her total being, the being that she was. That just baffles me. Did we miss something. Did we not see something that was coming on or what?

ANNE: What do you mean?

MARITA: Well, usually if somebody is deteriorating you can note something. You could distinctly tell that something is wrong. But we never picked it up. We tried to pick at it the other day like did we miss something. Was she coming to this day where she would forget to eat? She forgot that she was hungry. She forgot that she had to urinate.

ANNE: Before, would she be able to tell you if she needed to go to the bathroom?

MARITA: Well, she would be incontinent. It was just the idea. She would still be looking for the bathroom even though she was incontinent. What happened? What jarred her?

ANNE: Are you suggesting that there's something other than the fall that's happening here?

MARITA: Yea, it has to be because we know that the Alzheimer's have a different pain threshold. Sometimes they will feel the pain. Other times they'll walk around with a broken hip or it's newly broken or a recent surgery and they'll walk around like it's nothing. But the majority of the time they forget. They appear to feel the pain. But this was a fracture on her. It had nothing to do with the mental state. But then all of a sudden, why did this occur? When her pubis fractured, her mind went too, it seemed like to me.

The next day, the staff's spirits were lifted. Justine expresses their protection and then release of Marge to hospice,

> We have had a shield around her. When the hospice people would come we would always watch them. We didn't want to say well you're not doing this right because everybody does things differently. But we had a kind of shield. We had to put that shield away so that they could care for her as well. We felt that if she stayed with us that she would be alright.[10]

By the end of the week the mood among staff had changed to one of anger, grief and loss. The order came from the physician and director of nursing to move Marge to the non-ambulatory Third Unit. The staff gathered to reflect on this decision over which they had no control:

> ARNELLA: We all are depressed and angry at Marge being moved to non-ambulatory 3rd unit. We thought the administration was going to at least wait until we attempted to walk her again. They didn't give us a chance. They made the decision but I think they never attempted to solve the problem so they just threw her over there.
>
> CARMA: None of us wanted her to go because we felt that if she could stay with us she was going to be walking again.
>
> MARITA: Everybody is hurting and we are so mad. We cried because we were all sad that they would take her from us, although she's still on the same floor with us. But it's not like home, where on our side, it's home for her. We were quite upset because there was nothing we could do. We just had to grin and bear it.

For the staff, the loss of Marge is not only an intrusion and substantial emotional loss, but an ultimate loss of autonomy. Staff work in the shadow of the third unit whose doors remain shut at all times. Rarely mentioned, the third unit houses dementia patients who are non-ambulatory and receive palliative care. To the CNAs, it symbolizes death.[11]

Notes

1 As I talked with CNAs, I began to hear the phrase "getting into the resident's world" over and over again. "Getting into the resident's world" is a situationally grounded skill whereby the staff orient to, and learn to use, residents' own understandings and meanings of what is going on. While the entire interaction between staff and residents in this book exemplifies different ways that the staff attempt to get into the resident's world, I address the phenomenon conceptually in this chapter within the continuing narrative. There are two overarching aims employed in this important skill: (a) meeting the emotional needs of residents and preserving dimensions of resident self and mind; and (b) assisting staff to discern where the resident is to convince the resident to "go along" with certain staff concerns.

2 This exchange summons identity and continuity with a former social position and occupational identity of the two men. The meeting may also be interpreted as an invitation from Ben and Mr. Randolph to LPN Marita to join their world and to participate in the construction of a self (the occupational self, the resourceful self who has a certain province over money and friendship). Ben is prevailing upon Marita to act on the friendship role. Both men have challenged Marita to enter a collaborative construction of selves. In so doing, she acknowledges agency and authenticates being. Marita's strategy serves her *own* needs in this situation to get relief from residents' requests on this subject. Marita told me later that the meeting was soon forgotten because the next day it was a "whole different world." She said, however, "Sometimes I confuse myself by 'stepping in' because you can't step out of it right away. You cannot. I had to sit back there for a while and get my grip before I could go back to the desk." Her words convey a move into a finite province of meaning, which is also a depletion of Marita's energy. These are not uncomplicated exchanges even though they may appear to be. Marita's creative move to the back area of the Pavilion for the meeting reinforces the serious purpose of a *business* meeting where alternative worlds can be constructed for the residents. Using the residents' meaning of the situation to construct a situation helps direct their energies at that precise time. It may provide satisfaction for Boris to have acted out his role of businessman and his role of emotional attachment to Carrie Mae. She in turn has an opportunity to express her point of view even in the face of some disdain from Boris Randolph. We have no way of knowing how Carrie Mae feels about her position within this threesome. Marita Martin's earlier interpretation of Carrie Mae's relationship with Boris Randolph suggests a subservient role.

3 Justine begins by asking questions and reaching out to Miss Ava so that she can get her to go to bed. She offers choices of action to Ava, for example, doing puzzles, getting something to eat, or smoking a cigarette or working. These activities provide the possibility for shared experience. CNA Justine engages Miss Ava in action that sets up a reciprocity of the *capability* to care—giving and receiving a back rub, an intimacy. In this scenario, Miss Ava becomes an agent. The mutual neck rubbing and taking turns are acts of significance having consequences for future relations with the resident. These small, cumulative acts that Justine contributes to and shares with Ava had the effect of eventually putting her "out" as Justine describes it. Justine and Ava shared an experience with each other in a "bare bones" way in the canteen over a cigarette, letting their hair down together. In contrast to CNA Glenda, who "gets on the same level with Miss Ava" through matching her shouting louder and louder, Justine gets on the same level with Ava from a different set of assumptions that allow Ava to "use her mind." Both CNAs have similar intentions; they take what they interpret are the resident's ways of understanding as the conduit to their world. In the end, what may allow for more resolution is Justine's long-term relationship with Aunt Ava.

4 As reflected in Glenda's comments, the staff view the resident's world as very much a place, what I call "destinations of the mind." They attempt to be "in place," to be on common *emotional* and geographic ground with the resident. The staff set out to accomplish this "being with" the resident in her or his own world through dialogue, listening, or through action.

5 Philosopher, sociologist and social behaviorist, George Herbert Mead, explains the origin of mind and self and identifies the mechanism by which mind and self arise within the basic social process of communication. For Mead, self and society are "twin-born"; the self evolves through various stages from infant to adulthood in the all-important context of society; the self is active, not passive; and, humans communicate through symbols. Mead emphasized how critical language is to the whole endeavor of communication

and socialization. For our purposes in this research, parts of Mead's work can help to illuminate the complexity of the attempts of the staff to communicate with residents. We have popularized the *technique* of "role-playing" for various purposes, but *taking* the role of the other is something altogether different, something deeper than applied technique. According to Mead, *Mind, Self and Society: From the Standpoint of a Social Behaviorist* (Chicago, IL: University of Chicago Press, 1934: 327, 286–287), "The development of communication is not simply a matter of abstract ideas, but is a process of putting one's self in the place of the other person's attitude." For Mead, attitudes encompass both verbal and nonverbal aspects. He defines them (within interaction) as "stages in the act as they appear to others—expressions of countenance, positions of the body, changes in breathing, outward evidence of circulatory changes, and vocal sounds." We have ample empirical evidence of staff's attempts at deep participation such as Mead is talking about. Justine's vivid description of "jumping" into the resident's world, whatever they're going through, "we have to get in there and we go through that with them" makes the point. Mead's theory, however, assumes at least the *capacity* for reciprocity between persons in communication, something which is fleeting and which the staff cannot count on with residents. Therefore, taking the role of the other in the presence of dementia must take place within the *framework* of "getting into the resident's world." Staff immersion in an individual resident's world may produce a kind of intermittent reciprocity between staff member and a resident. Negotiation between resident self and staff member and adjustment of each participant to what the other is saying and/or doing, may, at least, allow for fragments of shared meaning and the emergence of dimensions of resident self. The question becomes how might this process enhance emotional well-being and help preserve aspects of resident self?

6 Whether there is a persisting self in the presence of dementia is a subject of debate among researchers. Lisa Caudell and Linda Clare, "The Impact of Dementia on Self and Identity," *Clinical Psychology Review* 20 (2010): 113–126, present a comprehensive review of the literature indicating that differences exist on a continuum. On one end are researchers who believe that the self remains throughout the course of dementia: Sam Fazio and David B. Mitchell, "Persistence of Self in Individuals with Alzheimer's Disease," *Dementia* 8 (2009): 39–59. In the middle of the continuum are researchers who suggest that a "compromised" self remains to a certain degree: Jiska Cohen-Mansfield, Aleksandra Parpura-Gill and Hava Golander, "Salience of Self-Identity Roles in persons with Dementia: Difference in Perceptions among Elderly Persons, Family Members, and Caregivers," *Social Science and Medicine* 62 (2006): 745–757, and D. Addis and L. Tippett, "Memory of Myself: Autobiographical Memory and Identity in Alzheimer's Disease," *Memory* 12 (2004): 56–74. At the other end of the continuum is the contention that the self is destroyed by the disease as argued by Daniel Davis, "Dementia: Sociological and Philosophical Constructions," *Social Science and Medicine* 58 (2004): 369–378.

In his in-depth research over the last twenty years, psychologist Steven Sabat has found that self, "the self of personal identity, persists far into the end stage of the disease." For more detail on his work see Steven Sabat and Rom Harre, "The Construction and Deconstruction of Self in Alzheimer's Disease," *Aging and Society* 12 (1992): 443–461. See also Steven Sabat and Michelle Collins, "Intact Social, Cognitive Ability, and Selfhood: A Case Study of Alzheimer's Disease," *American Journal of Alzheimer's Disease* 14 (1999): 17. In his book, *The Experience of Alzheimer's Disease: Life Through a Tangled Veil* (Malden, MA: Blackwell Publishers, 2001), Sabat criticizes the common way that persons with Alzheimer's disease are "assessed" through quantitative methods to measure their cognitive dysfunction which does not take into account understanding the whole person. He talked with men and women who have been diagnosed with probable Alzheimer's disease and described their disillusionment and powerlessness as it affected their quality of life and sense of self. He advocates for an approach that restores a sense of pride in persons with Alzheimer's. The difficulty surrounding research into the perpetuation of self is due to varying definitions of self and the research methodology (qualitative or quantitative) used in the studies; however, the critical point is *how* positions on self in the presence of dementia affect the *practice* of care work with what consequences. Regarding the existence and preservation of resident's self-identity, also see Renée Beard, "In Their Voices: Identity Preservation and Experiences of Alzheimer's Disease," *Journal of Aging Studies* 18 (2004): 415–428, and Pia Kontos, "Ethnographic Reflections on Selfhood, Embodiment and Alzheimer's Disease," *Aging and Society* 24 (2004): 829–849.

7 Marita Martin and the CNAs have a positive valence on resident self. They recognize and act toward dimensions of individual, idiosyncratic resident self *even while* they do so within a broader framework in which the residents are viewed as partially disabled. Yet, alongside that view exists the CNAs' refrain of residents "using their minds" and daily efforts to arouse self and mind as part of their care. The primacy of that endeavor in the CNAs' care work is evident when Marita Martin emphasizes that, "The most important thing is to keep their self." CNA Justine expresses it in these terms,

> I enjoy doing with them what they like to do. Because to me, when they do something that they've been doing or are used to doing, then they're using their mind. They say Alzheimer's but then they're thinking for themselves. They are doing it. And I like that.

Justine attributes thinking, a kind of "mindedness" to residents, to "know that mind is steady working." As well, other CNAs speak of "keeping up the resident's self-esteem" as a daily task.

How are we to make sense of what might appear to be a contradiction between assumptions about a resident's limited competence and the importance CNAs place on residents' ability to use their minds? First, persons and groups can hold simultaneously "divergent currents" or thoughts. Furthermore, as human beings, it is rare *not* to hold contradictory thoughts and feelings even if we choose not to recognize or publicly acknowledge them. In *Conflict and The Web of Group Affiliation* (New York: The Free Press, 1955: 15–17), Georg Simmel asserts that "… a pure unification not only is empirically unreal, it could show no life process." Second, what we may view as ironic can contain within it a "mindful decision" on the part of CNAs. For example, CNA Carma speaks of a deliberate disposition toward the residents when she first came to the Alzheimer's Pavilion: "I decided I was going to have respect for the individual. I was going to *treat them like they were whole*. If they progress one inch that's everything to me." From the staff's perspective, complete loss of self is not *inevitable*, not *absolute* during the course of a resident's time on the Pavilion. Various parts of self survive. Third, to further complicate the staffs' position on resident self, we must allow for both a cognitive self and an affective self. The CNAs' desire to refute *common assumptions* of "no-self" is strong. Marita and her staff can end up evoking several *dimensions* of self (occupational self, emotional self, social-class self, gendered self, racial self, creative self and so forth). The staff are aware of the conceptions of the medical model of inevitable, progressive degeneration; however, they tend to relate to the residents as though this were not a certainty and do what they can to slow the pace of the progression, dreading when residents, as staff say, "take a turn."

8 The meaning of control in this situation is to accomplish a task and to honor the family's request. Control of the situation and supporting the emotional well-being of Mary Louise are Marita's primary objectives. Skills of this kind require much energy, time, concentration, presence and respect. Yet, such skills are *never* captured in the official chart. Marita communicates with Mary Louise primarily through non-symbolic interaction, based on her knowledge of the other through touch, eye contact, countenance and rhythm. Communication is multidimensional, is not only cognitive but also affective. In a logico-deductive world of scientific inquiry we give minimal attention (or none at all) to the equally important emotional content of interactive exchange. Herbert Blumer, "Social Attitudes and Nonsymbolic Interaction," *Journal of Educational Sociology* 9 (1936): 517, follows Mead and elaborates: "Feeling is intrinsic to every social attitude—it is not to be treated as an additional element fused into some symbolic structure ..." He identifies "two phases of attitudes: (1) a symbolic aspect and, (2) an affective aspect assuring the attitude its liveliness, its movement, its vigor, and its tenacity." Mary Louise, *as far as we know*, cannot engage in verbal give and take based on the creation of shared meaning through cognitive (symbolic) interaction. How do we know what, or if, meaning has been created here? We do not know for sure but what we do know is the presence of the crucial element of *intention* on the part of Marita Martin to communicate and the need for a practical, positive outcome. In this case, Mary Louise, known for her volatility (sometimes extreme), is quieted so the task can be completed before her daughter arrives.

9 From the perspective of communication as multidimensional and multi-channeled, the series of selves can be viewed as a channel of communication. I view the series of selves in two ways: first, as *connecting points* through which the staff "reassure the resident of their well-being, and strive to communicate experientially with the residents, whatever it takes," as CNA Diane Allen puts it; and second, as *organizing points*, which staff use to enter the resident's world to control and bring about changes in behavior. The CNAs *evoke* and respond to the storied self and the new self in interaction with the residents. They *create* the imagined self through a collection of bits and pieces of the storied and new selves gleaned from resident narratives.

10 Noteworthy, on the one hand, are the staff's decision and Justine's choice of words regarding hospice, "We had to put that shield away so that they could care for her as well." In her preface to this remark, Justine makes sure that she articulates that the CNAs did their job first, "We would always watch them (hospice)" an indication and use of their autonomy to evaluate and "allow" hospice to come in, perhaps because their philosophy of care was more consonant with the CNAs' than not. On the other hand, the staff must make this choice if they want to keep Marge with them in the Pavilion, as Justine implies in her last line, "We felt that if she stayed with us she would be alright." Here lay the tensions between assertion of autonomy and compromise, the contested ownership of space between insiders and outsiders. Most important, however, is to recognize the subtle point embodied herein. The nature of the compromise is not having to *acquiesce* to the physician's "orders" as in the medical model of care but *making a choice* for care that resonates with their own. The use of the word "shield" connotes a combative stance as well as a protective one. Justine's remark to me one day comes to mind, "I don't care, I told Mr. Greenburg, I would lose my job if it meant protecting them (the residents)."

11 The late Tom Kitwood, *Dementia Reconsidered: The Person Comes First* (Buckingham: Open University Press, 1997: 8, 45), has provided some of the most brilliant work and theoretical discussion about care work for persons with dementia.

Kitwood defines personhood in the following way: "It is a standing or station that is bestowed upon one human being by others, in the context of relationship and social being. Both according of personhood, and the failure to do so, have consequences that are empirically testable." Kitwood warns the medical and social science communities against the use of a "malignant social psychology in caring for those diagnosed with dementia and probable Alzheimer's disease." He says:

> In care practice … whether in institutions or in the community, contains the residues of at least four depersonalizing traditions: bestialization, the attribution of moral deficit, warehousing, and the unnecessary use of a medical model. Among all fields, provisions for people who have dementia is perhaps the most affected because gross under-resourcing is compounded by fear, defense and a pervasive ageism.

4

SHARED MEANING AND IDENTITY WORK

On a warm Wednesday morning in April, as I head for a seat in the family room, I notice CNA Justine and Miss Ava Reynolds going into a resident's room. Their arms are loaded with fresh linens for the bed. Miss Ava looks very determined, is the leader in this activity, and is well "turned out" at this hour. In about fifteen minutes they both appear in the corridor, walk a few feet, turn, and enter another resident's room. Justine must be taking care of bed work; however, why is Miss Ava accompanying her in such an organized fashion? Just as I arrive, Justine thanks Aunt Ava for her help and they part company. I catch Justine's eye, "Miss Ava is in a good mood. What's up?" With a certain cadence, CNA Justine Jackson relates an example of what she calls "keeping busy with the residents" through the shared routine of making the beds with Miss Ava in the morning after breakfast. Here is her description of Ava Reynolds, a former domestic worker, making beds:

> Ava makes a mean bed. Square corners and everything. And she beats them pillows. So sometimes I tell them "Don't make the bed. Me and Ava going to do it." I say, "Come on girl, we've got so many beds." We go from room to room and we make them beds. But there's not a whole lot she'll let me do. I say, "Let me." "No," she says, "You go on over there. You do that. I've got this right here." And she's just in a good mood. And I like to see her doing that. It lets me know that mind is workin'. She's thinking. She's tuckin' them sheets. She makes a me...an bed.

In Justine's telling, one can sense a timing and colorfulness to the whole activity, thereby reconstructing the past in the present, responding to the occupational self and emotional needs of Aunt Ava. One of the purposes is to evaluate the cognitive capacities of the resident and focus Ava's considerable energy and fiery behavior. The unanticipated consequences are helpful to everyone because the beds are getting made and freeing other CNAs to respond to residents.

The Alzheimer's Pavilion at Starrmount Geriatric provides a unique organizational setting where staff have a fair amount of autonomy, allowing them the freedom to interpret and assign meanings and to recognize and attribute identities to themselves and residents. This is unusual in that low-level workers, whom one might expect in another setting to be highly regulated and supervised, in the Pavilion have an organizational structure where they can construct meaningful work. Managers seldom visit; they are insulated from the larger institution; no one wants to get close to this work. Much of the time, Pavilion staff employ their own frameworks of care, unchallenged. This autonomy stands in contrast to research reports from other notable nursing home studies. Moreover, it is key in explaining how the CNAs' meanings so clearly shape the Pavilion and mold an ethic of care in opposition to the more common, strictly routinized medical model.

Interpreting and Assigning Meaning

Just before lunch, Mr. Randolph, CNA Diane, and I take a walk. Mr. Randolph is dressed in a v-neck sweater and a button-down shirt, both of which are tucked into his pants. His fedora is perched just so on his head. Still possessed of a dapper manner, Boris Randolph makes sure to open the door for us to step from the Pavilion into the greenery of the courtyard. The unmistakable sound of crunching leaves accompanies each step. Boris comments, "they really ought to get all that stuff up. You know, my brother George came here and took care of it." "What kind of work was George in?" asks Diane. "I just couldn't say." We stop by a modern sculpture, "The Spirit of Job". Mr. Randolph reads the dedication and pronounces Job as in work. After about ten minutes we arrive at the door to come inside. Residents do not come out to the courtyard by themselves. On most occasions, a CNA or family member comes along to manage the door. But today, Boris uses all of his strength to pull open the door for Diane and me as the interlude comes to an end.[1]

There are many sides to Mr. Randolph. As we say adieu to him, I remember an incident that happened one afternoon the week before. A vigorous exchange was going on between Boris and Diane concerning his closet door. "Why is this door locked?" demands Mr. Randolph. "It's locked to protect your stuff," answers Diane. "When I see security I will talk with them about it to see if they can open it for you. But right now it's locked." Boris continues to examine his closet door. A few minutes pass and in an angry tone he asks Diane again, "Why is my door LOCKED?"

Diane explains that she understood what would have meaning for Boris in this situation:

> I put a note on his door: *"Your closet is locked for security reasons, to protect your things. When I see a man in security we will talk to him about unlocking your closet."* I put on there: *"The Management."* That's his lingo. That's how he understands things—I put them under management. Now with somebody else you might put a family member. It just depends on their understanding of things. You have to step into their world and get into the way they're thinking.

Diane attempts to reassure Mr. Randolph and to use language that invokes his occupational identity; she is betting on his positive response to the authority behind the note. Her purpose is to appeal to Boris's rational self and lessen his emotional valence which, if not controlled, can snowball to other residents.

Another of the many examples of assigning meaning[2] to resident's actions comes from LPN Marita Martin and concerns residents Carrie Mae Gordon and Boris Randolph, who are good friends, and Ava Reynolds. One morning CNAs were giving Carrie Mae a bath and they noticed she had bruises on her back and they looked like hits. Marita had known Mr. Randolph to hit Carrie and she planned to ask about the bruises that afternoon to see if Carrie Mae remembered them. Marita tells me, "She didn't remember the bruises until I touched her back and they were sore. Then it clicked. I said, 'Why do you let him hit you?' Carrie said, 'Oh, my brother's like that. He likes to play rough.'"

ANNE: So you didn't ask her if she'd been hit. You asked, "Why do you let him hit you?"

MARITA: It was like she couldn't remember. It took me a while for her to understand what I was saying so I touched back there and it was, "Oh, he plays rough with me—my brother." That day it was her brother. The one thing I could get out of her was she was compliant. She was submissive to him no matter what he did. It's ok. It's ok for him to do this to me. You know what that told me? This is the way she was. She's very subservient. She couldn't even complain if she wanted to. She just kept it inside. That why I think that the anger in these people—in the age group that I'm taking care of—it's good for them to get mad because this has been repressed. This is anger that needs to come out. With Mr. Randolph, being the banker that he was, he repressed a lot of stuff. I bet he wanted to tell some people off so bad but he couldn't because he was in a position where he had to control his behavior. It had to be so-so.

ANNE: Are you suggesting that reasons for the anger of some residents comes from past experiences that we may or may not know about?

MARITA: Yes, I think a lot of times when they do get angry this is repressed anger because it could be the simplest things and they become angry.

ANNE: So there is a reason for the anger?

MARITA: Ava Reynolds is a good example. She is a black woman who is cleaning rooms and who has white bosses (in the past). She doesn't like having anyone tell her what to do.

ANNE: In her work or in anything?

MARITA: In anything. I think a lot of this is an overlapping of when they were young and what they have been repressing. So whenever that anger comes out ... you know they might be justified in being angry but the majority of the time it is something simple but you have to consider she is a woman who is cleaning an eight-story building. Then she became the supervisor and she became the boss. She has so much anger in her. The slightest thing just sets her off and you know the only one who can control that is Justine.

Marita grew up with a mother who worked on a "psych ward" and she herself worked on a hospital psychiatric ward, both of which may have nurtured her psychological acumen.

"Let them Sleep on the Couch"

On a cold Tuesday morning in late October, I arrive on the Pavilion around 6:30 am and find residents Martin Lovett sleeping on one couch and Alice Daly asleep on the other couch in the sitting room. RN Elaine Pressley is standing by the nurse's alcove. "What on earth are you doing here at this hour," she calls to me. "Just seeing if there is anything exciting going on around here," I say. We both laugh. "We...lll," Elaine says, referring to the residents asleep on the couch, "traditional, by-the-book nurses would *DIS*-approve of any resident sleeping overnight outside of their rooms." Such (public) freedom and out-of placeness would be unacceptable. The norms on the Alzheimer's Pavilion conflict with the norms of traditional nursing techniques designed to maintain order. Pressley continues,

> We have some wonderful nurses here at Starrmount but some of them are hyper. They'd have all the patients off the ceiling. They'd rush around and say, "We have to get this done. Have to get that done." No you don't.

Pressley will not let CNAs who are "rigid" work on the Pavilion.[3]

At this time of day, the Pavilion is filled with quiet. Arnella and Glenda are folding resident clothing and sorting laundry, a never-ending, frustrating task. Mr. Lovett stirs a bit on the couch, opens his eyes and smiles at me. I wave, note his unmatched socks, chuckle to myself, and head around by the fish tank to take a seat. I want time to think more about what Marita Martin asked me yesterday and to talk with her again today about the "aura." Several residents are peripatetic walkers. Boris Randolph, life-long bachelor who dresses well, saunters. Fay Morgan and Mabel Turner, both former teachers, tend to glide along the corridor as though they are ice skating (although that can change to frantic searching now and then) while trying to avoid Marge Jacobs who is doing her usual two-step dance. Staff refer to these resident movements as "being busy." Samuel Gold has just arrived for respite care. Moving up the corridor like a man on a mission, he creates a bit of a stir, his cane thumping hard on the linoleum floor keeping time with his strident gait as he heads for "his" big chair in the sitting area. For Henrietta Stein, Martin Lovett and Ruby Klein, ownership of space in the sitting area is very important and may lead, in the case of Henrietta Stein, to confrontations with both staff and residents.

At this hour, the sitting area is empty except for Irene and Martin. As I watch and listen to the birth of another day on the Pavilion, a substitute aide pulled from another floor comes over and joins me on the bench. She is waiting to meet with Marita Martin to get her assignment for the day. Jen has a ten-year background as a CNA, one year of that at Starrmount on the second floor of the nursing home. She tells me about her experiences as a substitute every now and then on the Alzheimer's Pavilion revealing how "difference" can be disparaging:

JEN: The disease, it's awful, it's the worst thing in the world to lose your mind. There are some pretty ladies down there and some of 'em aren't even that old. Oh … to lose your mind—it's awful, worse than AIDS … nothing like it … Why, they could be out doing things, being productive if they had their minds. It just is so sad.

ANNE: Is sadness something you feel when you are here?

JEN: Well, yes I guess it is. What could be worse? Don't get me wrong. I know they can't help it and I wish they were well but (she takes her hands and waves them in a sweeping gesture downward with much intensity). I've told them but they don't believe me. They will when something happens (ominous tone) (I) can't stand people wandering around all the time, putting their hands on you. They *kiss* each other (said with distaste). They come up and say, "Boo!" Can't stand it! Or, going around and wiping tables and everything in sight. It's a crazy, looney bin (nervous laugh). I shouldn't say that.

ANNE: Working here is different?

JEN: Well it HAS to be (shouting). Working on the third floor people know what they are doing. They have their mental faculties and you can tell them something and they know. Here you have to say "come give me this, don't do that, stay over here." It's like baby sitting and I forget sometimes that I am baby sitting and then, boy something can happen.

ANNE: Like what?

JEN: I lasted thirty days on an Alzheimer's Unit elsewhere. Then I went looney.

ANNE: Do they know you feel this way?

JEN: No.

ANNE: What about the staff?

JEN: They're very mellow down here. Different than up on my floor. Don't think we (3rd floor) could have the patience.

ANNE: What would be a good day on the Pavilion?

JEN: When I don't get any back talk.

ANNE: How did you feel when you left the other day?

JEN: Boy, I'm glad this is over. It is easier here because you don't have to turn or lift patients … but oh … the *mental.*

ANNE: Have you ever felt fear?

JEN: Oh, yes. They fight you if you don't watch out and if they don't want something. Like to put on a bib. And then one day, a man I didn't know who was a resident was at the door and wanted out. He put his hand out to hit me because I wouldn't let him out. I have no patience. I'm good at what I do (laughs). But I don't like to get close to anyone (emphasizes with feeling and intensity). I don't like to talk and I would have to on the Alzheimer's Pavilion.

ANNE: Would you have to get close to the residents?

JEN: What is there to get close to? There's nothing there (referring to the residents). All that touching and sounds and moving around all over the place. I don't like people moving all around me, all over the place.

Our conversation ends when LPN Marita calls Jen over for the day's assignment.

What is so distasteful to the substitute aide is the essence of the staff's approach at the Helen Wise Alzheimer's Pavilion. The philosophy and guiding principles of the Pavilion grew out of a partnership between the social services department and the nursing department at Starrmount Geriatric. Elaine Pressley, RN, Head Nurse, sums it up when she comments that she and Carol Stanforth, head of social services, had "a lot of the same feeling about the freedom to let people be, and to improve the quality of their life." The staff wish to adapt the environment to the resident, not the resident to the environment. In stark contrast to substitute CNA Lisa's perspective, RN Elaine Pressley speaks of the heart of that philosophy, which is:

> to make it home-like for them and a place where they will be contented and know that they don't have to conform, that they can do their own thing. They don't have to go to bed. Let them sleep on the couch. You can't get uptight because somebody doesn't want to do something when you want them to do it. Maybe their room doesn't look like you think it should look. But if they've messed it up it's immaterial. I've learned from experience that certain things aren't important. Making residents' lives more meaningful and enjoyable is more important than worrying about is the bed made or the covers aren't tight. That's nice to look at but that doesn't make the residents' lives better. "We mostly do things by feel down here," she tells me.

Recognizing and Attributing Identities (Identity Work)

On a morning just before Thanksgiving, the atmosphere in the Pavilion is leisurely and serene. Residents are dozing a bit after breakfast, but not for long. Marita

Martin has just put on some music and CNAs are going from room to room, cleaning up and sorting clothing. The maintenance crew has cleared the dining area and the slow bossa nova music curls itself around the room. CNA Glenda walks over and extends her hands to residents Jenny and Belle to invite them onto the dance floor. For the size of Glenda, she has an easy glide with her feet and a practiced touch as her arched and extended arms connect with Jenny and Belle in a circle of dance. Jenny is radiant as she does an easy two-step, as is Belle. All are as light as air. Glenda's countenance is tender at this moment with a shy innocence as well as an easy comfortableness. She has brought them into her element as she invites them to move as she moves. Jenny watches Glenda's feet. Smiling, Glenda says to them, "You were gooood." There is no mistaking the enjoyment and what seems a quiet pride. Time is not so harsh at this moment for these three.

With a load of laundered clothes in her arms, CNA Carma Lee passes by the dance scene and calls to Ruby Klein who is approaching with her walker, "Hi lil' sister. How are you feelin' this morning." "You're looking stronger, Miss Vogue," says Glenda as she gives Ruby a hug. When I ask Carma later if she were aware of calling Ruby "lil' sister" she responds with, "Was that me?" Carrie Mae, fascinated by the dance scene, attempts a move into the gliding and prancing of Lily, already firmly ensconced on the dance floor. Marita calls to Carrie Mae, "Hey, grandma, let's watch from over here on the side. This is Lily's show now." Carma Lee mentioned to me that Lily's daughter came in one day when her Mother was dancing and exclaimed, "I never saw or knew that Mother could dance!" It was a shocking surprise but a pleasing one for the daughter who had known her mother as self-composed, not given to public displays of such obvious enjoyment and individual expression. Staff's encouragement of free creative expression also enlarges the identity of Belle as they think of her as the dancer along with Jenny.

During my many hours of observation at Starrmount, there were few times of total quiet on the Pavilion. Engagement between staff and residents with other residents was a given. The exception was "quiet time," developed by Marita Martin, which took place just before lunch when lights were turned off or low for a specified period of time. In contrast, Diamond describes the spaces with residents in the nursing homes he studied as "rooms filled with quiet. Forty women and ten or twelve men sat assembled together, not talking."[4]

Some might argue that vocal behavior is spurious behavior only, not meaningfully directed behavior appropriate to time and place. Much of the time, however, the staff did not treat such behavior as spurious but related to another construction that required they enter to understand, be present in, or redirect the behavior. Maybe you would think this was errant behavior of some of the residents purportedly attributed to dementia and descriptions of "acting out." No question, there were multiple realities operating here and that was the challenge for the staff who had to move in and out of those realities. But … there was also laughter, dancing and spontaneous singing. That was because of the levels of autonomy that the CNAs had—the TIME they had to create schedules, albeit interrupted at times.

Also, they had the time to "do family,"[5] that is, they construct family through language and emotional connection; they act toward and speak to the residents as family, as extended kin. The CNAs reproduce a version of alternate kin that arises out of black culture. Arnella explains how "doing" family is accomplished:

> The staff and the residents, we try to be more like a family, all of us, you know. We talk to each other like we're family—sister, aunt, grandma, grandpa, uncle, girlfriend. We hug, you know, we are affectionate with the people, the staff and residents. You see someone that needs a hug, not only do we hug the residents, they hug each other. They know when something's wrong with one of the others. They question you just like family. We are totally different from all the other units.

LPN Marita adds:

> Well, number one, you know that when you are there for an individual, you need the nurturing. The person needs that nurturing. It's like we are family. I don't think I can say anything else. We're a family, we're a unit. I'm not saying unit as in a ward. I'm saying unit as in a family. We all have these roles to play. I think we hit it on the nose when we gather with them. They love touch.

There is a blurring of the lines between family and friends. Friends also become family. Staff's behavior over several months suggests that the identity of residents incorporates a complex mix of adult and child[6] with an important distinction: *talking about* them and *behaving toward* them. The majority of staff state: "Be calm with them and don't treat them like babies. They're not babies. They're adults and be clear with them." Justine adds, "First of all we're all adults here. We don't have a sense of ordering them around. We just don't do that." At the same time, when talking about the residents to me they would refer every once in a while to residents as "leaving their kids," "the residents being in their terrible twos," and "protecting them like they were our kids."

The intermingling of constructing family and attributing personal identities such as "Miss Vogue," (a nickname for Ruby because she likes to "look pretty" and has fashionable clothes), keeps unique identity traits of residents before the staff. They are claimed and reinforced by being spoken aloud as part of everyday interaction.

Employing Their Own Frameworks

> *Words sculpt the lifeworld of the Pavilion into patterns and practices that hold tight and then release the fragile, yet persisting self of the resident, like breathing in and breathing out sustains life.*

As sounds diminish almost to a hush, my eyes travel to the second dining table where CNA Arnella is preparing to help Mary Catherine eat her lunch. They seem to be in their own time and motion sphere. There is a concentration in this act on the part of both. Arnella angles the spoon to go in the mouth and slides it in and up in unison with the movement of Mary Catherine's mouth, as though they both know the choreography of the moment. Then, any food left on the chin is gathered up by hand and spoon and whisked into the mouth. A quieter moment, a brief pause in the middle of the day.

It is about 1:45 pm now and the CNAs have been in and out of resident rooms toileting and readying the residents for the afternoon. CNA Chevelle and Roy are in conversation at the end of the row of dining tables, talking about Roy's wife. He is telling her that his wife is recovering from heart trouble. I take a seat at the end of the first dining table, my back to the courtyard where I can hear rain beating against the large windows. Abe Steck and LPN Marita are in conversation nearby:

MARITA: Well, Abe, couldn't you have spoken to someone else?

ABE: No, it had to be you because you sit with me and don't stare off some place. I was sitting over there by the table … and I had something I wanted to ask you, but I started thinking, they were confusing me. The words were confusing me. The words were confusing. Something's wrong with me.

MARITA: Why do you think that something is wrong with you?

ABE: (hesitating) Because … when I saw you, I knew your name but I couldn't say it. I wanted to ask questions and I know my words don't … come out so you can understand me.

MARITA: You know, see all these people sitting around (pointing to the sitting room)?

ABE: Yes.

MARITA: You know, they have the same problem, only yours isn't as bad as theirs is. Do you understand me?

ABE: I think I do. Are *you* like this?

MARITA: Well, sometimes I am. Sometimes I forget and sometimes I get rambled when I want to say something. Or, I'm ahead of myself and when I get ahead of myself, I can't express myself very well.

ABE: You've hit it on the nose, kid. Look at me. I need something, but I'm ashamed to ask. I woke up this morning and I didn't have my billfold.

At that moment, Marita is paged over the intercom for a meeting upstairs. Abe realizes that she has to go. "Thank you for listening to me. You've got a great smile." Marita smiles back and heads upstairs. I too must leave for the day, and say goodbye to resident Grace and her "community of neighbors." Marita Martin is standing at the elevator. I ask her about the conversation with Abe Steck. She had not chosen to put a name to the problem. She replied, "No, I didn't want to do that to him right now. I don't even know if I would ever label him."[7]

Marita Martin carefully crafts her words in interaction with Abe Steck. She avoids premature medical classification of Abe's symptoms. She makes an inclusive statement in *implying* that there can be a continuum of confusion in articulating one's thoughts ("I get rambled and ahead of myself sometimes when I am trying to say something"). She also speaks of *degrees along that continuum* when comparing his confusion with his fellow residents of the Pavilion. Marita conveys, fully, her understanding of his concerns and brings about possible clarity on Abe Steck's part; however, she does not *deny* Abe's anxiety and concerns. Staff strive for a distinct separation of the person and the disease when they can. So-called illness symptoms of Alzheimer's disease that are considered deviant and disruptive to orderly social life (inside and outside the institution) are attributed to the disease when CNAs defend the resident's behavior to family or outsiders who do not understand. Attribution is used as an explanation for protection of the person, not as corroborative evidence/legitimation of the status of the Alzheimer's patient. What are indicators of disease to some tend to become what I call "traits of being" to the staff because they want to salvage a self that they believe survives in spite of the disease.

Marita's explanation for the way she chose to respond to Abe reflects both a refined knowledge of residents and their circumstances as well as strategic thinking regarding what stance to take in relation to them. The fact that I found staff routinely employing complex knowledge and analytic thinking in their care work at Starrmount is highly significant because it contradicts previous studies which suggest that care work in nursing home settings consists largely of emotion-based as opposed to cognitively grounded responses. An important contribution of this book is to point out that the knowledge base accrued by frontline workers in these care settings has been neglected in favor of their emotional contributions.[8]

The elevator doors open, we say our goodbyes and I head for the main doors of Starrmount, thinking all the while of the importance of identity work among another group: the CNAs themselves.[9]

"It's Like a Finger's Missin'": Becoming a Team

It's Tuesday morning and baths are underway around 9:30 am. I can hear Henrietta in the whirlpool room as the CNAs are giving her a bath. Many residents dislike bathing in the whirlpool and are afraid of it. Henrietta is no exception; she is screaming at the top of her lungs:

HENRIETTA: Don't. Don't now, I don't need my hair washed, it's alright. Goddam you, Black bitch. (Silence) They used to have nice people here. Don't do that. No, no. Don't do that to my hair. Can't you be nicer?

AIDE: I'm as nice as I'm gonna be.

HENNIE: Oh, you HURT me.

Each CNA carries out no more than two baths per day. Baths are points of anxiety for the residents and may take anywhere from thirty to forty minutes or longer, depending on how much bathing is involved. To assure safety, a few residents are given baths in their room. Baths are staggered so that a couple of the CNAs are left in the living/sitting area to oversee activities such as reading to the residents and question and answer time, before the activities leader arrives. At the same time, laundry may arrive. According to staff, laundry duty is one of the most time-consuming, frustrating aspects of bed and body work: time-consuming because all the residents' clothes are mixed together, taken away and washed by a contractor, and when returned, the staff have to sort it for each resident; frustrating because the time the laundry arrives back on the unit varies from one day to the next. Simultaneously, the certified medication technician (CMT) dispenses medication to the residents. The Alzheimer's Pavilion at Starrmount has the least individuals on medication compared to the other floors of the facility, a fact that pleases Charge Nurse Marita Martin.

On this day in August, Carrie Mae has just received her medication from CNA Justine. Knowing her destination, she heads toward Boris Randolph, gives him a beguiling smile as she passes, and nestles herself into the chair next to him. According to the staff, they are "an item," that is, friends who "feel romantic toward each other." If the door to Mr. Randolph's room is closed, the CNAs do not intrude. Gathered outside the nurse's alcove, CNAs are talking about a wedding two of them attended over the weekend and how the dresses "weren't all white like traditional weddings a long time ago but more colors." With a sly grin on her face, one CNA wonders "how long it would last, knowing the two people" and everyone explodes in laughter. LPN Marita Martin is working on resident charts inside the alcove when she is jarred to her feet by the deafening sounds of chairs being yanked off the long dining table, thrown on the floor, and then slapped back onto the top of the table, one by one. The source of the mayhem is Miss Ava Reynolds who is "hoppin' mad." No one, not even the male janitor, can stop her except CNA Justine. Marita Martin shouts to the other CNAs, "Go get Justine right now. She'll know what to do. Miss Ava is out of control!" Then, as quickly as she began, Miss Ava comes to a halt and saunters away. Had Justine been there she would have tried speaking and listening to Miss Ava to "see where she was coming from." Justine is more attuned to Ava, and the staff depend on her when all else fails with Ava Reynolds.

The consistent message from Marita Martin and the CNAs is that they are an inter-dependent team, that their care work is a collective effort. One aspect of teamwork is the ability to sense when one member is nearing the end of her rope under the stress of multiple demands. On more than one occasion, I have watched Justine, second in command to LPN Marita, keeping her eye pealed for mounting stress in her co-workers. Justine detects such a state in CNA Carma Lee in the following:

Everyone is waiting for lunch. CNA Chevelle looks over at me and says in an anxious tone, "Waiting, waiting, waiting for lunch. Everyone is waiting for lunch." Carma has her hand on her head as though soothing her brow in the midst of the late arrival of lunch. All meals are to remain hot and must arrive a few at a time. Many residents are left without plates while they watch others eat. Resident complaints and questions about when they will eat come in a rush. CNAs attempt to quell the agitation by explaining the situation over and over to Ruby, Boris and Henrietta who tend to be the most vocal with the sharpest tongues. Except for Henrietta, most residents can be convinced to stay; only a few must be rounded up when their tray arrives. All residents remain on edge. The wait is interminable for Henrietta and she screams, "Bring us something good to eat and hurry up!" Ruby and resident Sally are circling the table, not wanting to sit. Roy and Boots are in animated conversation; others sit in quiet resignation. Resident Henrietta is very excited and calls out again for food, "Bring it down here. Come on and bring it down here." At that point, tired of the wait, Henrietta gets up from the table, hikes up her shoulders very straight, and marches toward the sitting room. No one stops her, not unusual given the complicated relationship the staff have with Henrietta Stein.

Right at that moment the fire alarm goes off. Resident Abe Levy has managed to open wide the door to the outside and stands on the threshold with one leg poised to take off. The cleaning woman shouts, "He kept saying he wanted to go home, to go home. I hope he doesn't hurt himself." CNA Carma Lee dashes toward the door just before Abe slips out of sight and brings him back into the Pavilion. CNA Justine's voice pierces across the room as she calls to CNA Carma Lee, "Hey, girl, come on and take a break. Go on, I'm here. What are you doin'? I'll finish it up. Take a break. Get away for a while." Carma Lee gives a hi-five sign and turns and heads out the door to the canteen for a short morning break. Justine motions to CNA Arnella and says,

> I'm goin' over to the third unit and if you need me holler. I'll be back. Just a matter of me turning that lock and sayin' I have to go back and help them. Arnella, lemme know if you want me to do the meds today.

Arnella calls back, "Ok and I'll help get Miss Ava up and then Glenda can get Marion up." Justine speaks of the solid center of staffs' relationship with each other: "There's something about us over here. We really have what's called teamwork. We stand behind each other. It's just like sisters."[10]

My observations of interaction on the Alzheimer's Pavilion and interviews with the staff demonstrate this perspective. The staff speak of getting support from each other on and off the Pavilion, looking out for one another, and possessing a strong loyalty to the group. In the following, Marita Martin captures the sentiments of the group when she speaks of unity in diversity:

> Teamwork. The chemistry. I let them know that we have a chemistry going. And they all agreed. They want to know why we work so good together. I said I'll think about it. We have oneness. We are a bunch of people with different personalities and different thoughts and different backgrounds and different education, but we're still one. I don't know how to express it verbally.

CNA Carma Lee puts it this way, "When someone's gone for a few days everything's kind of topsy turvy. It's the *whole association of the place* (my emphasis). If one is gone it's like a finger is missin'." Carma Lee's imagery is vivid, crystal clear and powerful in depicting the nature of teamwork on the Pavilion. Everything and everyone suffers when there is a substitute aide because the fingers of the hand are not complete and the hand is alien.

CNA Carma adds another dimension to the nature of teamwork on the Pavilion, knowing one's limitations and passing the task to another. Carma Lee does not like "reading to the residents" but enjoys "talking with them." She elaborates:

> The things that I know I can't handle I can delegate and let someone else do it. That helps me a lot. We kind of help each other. Things they don't like to do I usually like to do so it works out pretty good. I like the rotation because if you don't, Anne, you get into this routine of "Well this is my patient and no one can work like I do." That way you get a little taste of everybody. I like the rotation.

CNAs have eight residents each day for whom they are responsible and this constellation changes daily so that staff get to know all residents over a period of time. Carma Lee's insight into one of the personal gains from strong teamwork is noteworthy:

> With the right teamwork you can use other people as examples. Marita is a role model for me. I feel like I can talk to her if I'm having a problem. Arnella is pretty good. Like if I have a suggestion for the unit she is there. Always ready to do something new. If something isn't working we can find a solution, as a team. You have to feel that every resident is yours.

CNAs and Marita Martin express a feeling of solidarity against those outside their Pavilion. Justine speaks of an accord among the group that permeates all:

> There's a harmony. When one's hurting, we're all hurting. When one needs something … it's like a family. We all get into it together and take care of that problem. Whether it be on the job or off the job. You know when Marita was going through her little "thing" and we had planned a nice Christmas for her and everything so we waited and took care of her on her

> birthday when she was finally back with us. We were there for her. Whatever you need us to do just let us know. If you need a ride. Hey, I'll get a car and drive you to where you need to go. Don't worry, we're here.

When Justine talks about Marita's "little thing" she is referring to the short leave of absence that Marita took to deal with critical issues in her family. The Pavilion had a temporary Charge Nurse who was "not up to Marita Martin" according to the CNAs. To quote Elaine Pressley, "From the beginning Marita was 'a natural' for the Pavilion."

Sometimes, however, teamwork does not go well and may be thwarted by a member. Instead of being directed at facilitating care of the residents, team energy is diverted to another end. The CNAs might be having a "bad day" that needs to be straightened out before the staff go out on the Pavilion. If someone comes in depressed the staff will ask them about it; they need to "be at their best when they get out there with the residents," according to Marita Martin. One such occasion involved CNA Glenda and elicited a collective response from her co-workers:

> I think it was last Friday, I was real sick. What did I do? I came in and stayed in the bathroom all day vomiting. I got two people up. The rest, the co-workers helped me out. They made my beds for me. We were lucky we didn't have baths that day. They got people up for me. On other floors you don't have this (teamwork). You don't look for nobody to help. You don't look for nothing. No talking, no nothing. When people come down we communicate, we help. Marita let me sit and relax. But if that was another floor …

What Glenda fails to mention is the reason she was sick. She had a hangover. Marita Martin told me that she had "got on her" about it but that Glenda has a "good heart" and still has things to learn. Personal and family strife are ongoing concerns of the CNAs. Marita has screened calls for some CNAs to protect them from conversations with boyfriends and husbands who are alcoholics or "trouble-makers." It's not unusual that a teammate would take over duties for another member of the team. CNAs reinforce and construct a sense of cohesiveness through designation of "outsiders, those who do not understand the residents and all that we do," as Justine puts it.

At the same time that staff give examples of teamwork that is played out in covering duties for others and encouraging them to "take a break" off the Pavilion, the CNAs *do not want*, in practice, to take the breaks they are allowed and *required* to take by law. Avoiding breaks became such a problem that "an order from the top came down" that mandated scheduled breaks *outside the unit.* The CNAs' resistance to going off the Pavilion at prescribed times reveals something about the importance of worker control over their work. Required breaks are artificially inserted at points in time that may not correspond well with the flow of work on the Pavilion. CNAs are willing to take breaks on their *own* schedule, when necessary.

In his ethnography on institutional care, the daily lives of residents and aides, and the nursing home as industry, Timothy Diamond[11] broke new ground around the *relationship* between nursing aides and individual residents. While critically important, I argue that this insight is incomplete. Starrmount CNAs' quality of care work is embedded in, and arises out of, their relationship with residents but with one critical difference: care is also embedded in the relationship *among* the CNAs themselves, their *teamwork*. These two elements are inextricably bound because true teamwork is both relational and an essential part of the structure of the Pavilion.

For CNAs, the Pavilion is a refuge as well as a site of struggle. Anything but passive, these women and the LPN Charge Nurse work as a team to carry out the most demanding, soul-wrenching jobs at the bottom of the medical hierarchy. As workers, they defend and maintain their alternative care against formidable odds from families, administrative staff, physicians, and one of their own, a resident who flaunts her racism and classism. Henrietta Stein is the "hole" in their fabric of care work.

Notes

1 Even though Mr. Randolph can get mad at times and be incorrigible, he is recognized as a gentleman by all in the Pavilion. His dress (usually a coat and tie) and courtly manner, laced with a bit of dry wit, is apparent in his interaction with others. For his generation, the act of a male holding the door for a female was expected in terms of appropriate gendered behavior. Diane allows Boris Randolph to "do gender," that is, perform his culturally learned behavior thereby keeping intact one aspect of his identity which may serve as a reminder of that dimension of self. For more on doing gender, see Candice West and Don Zimmerman's classic article, "Doing Gender," *Gender and Society* 1 (1987): 125–151; and Judith Lorber, "Night to his Day: The Social Construction of Gender," in her *Paradoxes of Gender* (New Haven, CT: Yale University Press, 1995: 13–36).

2 Social research in medical care settings, Elliot Mishler et al., *Social Contexts of Health, Illness and Patient Care* (Cambridge, MA: Cambridge University Press, 1981: 198), suggests that cultural definitions and social meanings attached to illness, disability and aging have a powerful influence on the development and operations of care settings, as well as the social, behavioral and therapeutic processes occurring within these settings. George Herbert Mead, *Mind, Self and Society: From the Standpoint of a Social Behaviorist* (Chicago, IL: University of Chicago Press, 1934) emphasizes the ineluctable role of meaning in the formation of behavior. Human beings act on the basis of the meaning that objects in the environment have for them. For symbolic interactionists, meaning is not intrinsic to the object, but is assigned by the actor and always arises in social interaction within the life of human groups.

3 Elaine Pressley's words reflect the depth of the philosophy and guiding principles which emerged from developing the Pavilion. The CNAs worked to push the limits of freedom within the Alzheimer's Pavilion in the midst of the rationalized institution.

4 Diamond, Timothy. 1992. *Making Gray Gold: Narratives of Nursing Home Care*. Chicago, IL and London: University of Chicago Press.

5 For more on family as a socially constructed set of relationships, see Jaber Gubrium and David Buckholdt, *Fictive Family: Everyday Usage, Analytic, and Human Service Considerations* (Hoboken, NJ: Wiley-Blackwell, 1982: 878–885); Jaber Gubrium and James Holstein, *What is Family?* (Houston, TX: Mayfield Publishing, 1990: ix–x), in which they argue that the "everyday reality of the familial is produced through discourse. Thus, family is as much a way of thinking and talking … as it is a set of social ties and sentiments." Also see C. Berdes and J. Eckert, "The Language of Caring: Nurse's Aides' Use of Family Metaphors Conveys Affective Care," *The Gerontologist* 47 (2007): 340–349.

6 In contrast, Karen Lyman finds that CNAs mostly treat residents in adult day care as children. See Karen Lyman, "Infantilization of Elders: Day Care for Alzheimer's Disease Victims," in D. Wertz (ed.), *Research in the Sociology of Health Care* (Greenwich, CT: JAI Press, 1988: 71–103).

7 For insight on labeling and the medicalization of aging and dementia, see Carroll Estes and Elizabeth Binney, "The Biomedicalization of Aging: Dangers and Dilemmas," *The Gerontologist* 29 (1989): 587–596. Also see a classic article by K. Lyman, "Bringing the Social Back In: A Critique of the Biomedicalization of Dementia," *The Gerontologist* 29 (1989): 597–605. For more on a masculine-gendered experience of dementia, see Edward Tolhurst and Bernhard Weicht, "Preserving Personhood: The Strategies of Men Negotiating the Experience of Dementia," *Journal of Aging Studies* 40 (2017): 29–35.

8 In his ethnography, *Labors of Love: Nursing Homes and the Structures of Care Work* (New York: NYU Press, 2014: 18), Jason Rodriquez compares two nursing homes, one profit and one non-profit with regard to "the set of constraints and pressures that nursing home managers face from reimbursement and regulatory structures." Furthermore, he examines the "consequences of nursing home care in a way that is misaligned with the constraints" of such a system that is hierarchical, based on a medical model with no autonomy for frontline workers. Even though the focus of my research is different, I am interested in a central chapter in his book in which he discusses the "uses of emotion," which relates to my research at Starrmount. Rodriquez devotes a central chapter to the uses of emotion by nursing assistants to enhance their dignity and provide positive meaning to their demanding, devalued work. Also, he argues that emotional labor (care for a wage) was also a social control resource to get residents to do what the staff wanted them to do as a source of creating dignity and worth for the CNAs, a finding in my research; however, my research suggests that there is more to consider. I differ with Rodriquez in a fundamental way. Giving primacy to the uses of emotion in care work, for both nursing assistants and residents is not what I found. Starrmount CNAs used both cognition and emotion in their care work to garner a sense of their own worth and dignity, as well as to accomplish their ethic of care work with the residents. The problem is dichotomizing cognition and emotion from the beginning (the get-go). After many hours of observation and interviews with the CNAs and the LPN Charge Nurse, I was compelled to ground an understanding of their work from a position of first viewing them as sentient beings, as both conscious, cognitive and feeling beings. Humans are an amalgam of both. Theoretically, I chose to approach and understand the details of their work from that standpoint.

9 In "The Sociology of Feeling and Emotion: Selected Possibilities," published in an edited 1975 volume by Marcia Millman and Rosabeth Moss Cantor, entitled *In Another Voice: Feminist Perspectives on Social Life and Social Science*, (Garden City, NY: Anchor/Doubleday Press), Arlie Hochschild urges us to consider the image of the actor in social situations as a sentient actor (pg. 283). This article was written before she had developed her concept of "emotional labor." She comments (pg. 284)

> That … sociologists should attend to the actor's own definition of his or her feelings in order to find out how emotion vocabularies are used, what inner experiences they refer to, and what social situations call them forth or quash them.

Hochschild is right here, but she does not go far enough to be used in understanding care work. The CNAs' language of alternative care is a combination of cognition and feeling, which can revolutionize institutional and other forms of care. Related to my research, Steven Lopez, in his 2006 article, "Emotional Labor and Organized Emotional Care," *Work and Occupations* 33 (2): 136–160, discusses his concept of an alternative organizational strategy in nursing home care.

10 In their study of frontline workers, Robert Bogdan and Steven Taylor, "Let Them Eat Programs: Attendants' Perspectives and Programming in Wards in State Schools," *Journal of Health and Social Behavior* 15 (1974): 142–150, identify a "brotherhood at the bottom" among aides (low-level workers). These workers fraternize together, depend on one another and socialize off the job. The "sisterhood ensemble at the bottom" of Starrmount CNAs is similar to the affiliation among group members in that study. In her historical focus on values embedded in traditional African ancestry, Rosalyn Terborg-Penn, "Survival Strategies among African-American Women Workers: A Continuing Process," in Ruth Milkman (ed.), *Women, Work and Protest: A Century of U.S. Women's Labor History* (Boston, MA: Routledge & Kegan Paul, 2013: 139–155), emphasizes "the threads of continuity between ancestral African female traditions of mutual support and the self-organization of black women in contemporary society." Patricia Hill Collins, "Learning from the Outsider Within: The Sociological Significance of Black Feminist Thought," *Social Problems* 33 (1986): S25, writes in a similar vein but cautions us to remember that:

> There is no monolithic Black women's culture but a socially constructed Black women's culture. The particular nature of sisterhood is affected by the ancestral African-American traditions of mutual support but also takes on its own hue and social organization within the particular context out of which it arises.

Starrmount CNAs socially construct their own sisterhood with its particular "tone."

11 Timothy Diamond, *Making Gray Gold: Narratives of Nursing Home Care.* (Chicago, IL: University of Chicago Press, 1992: 166).

5

CO-CONSTRUCTING TROUBLE

> *"We all go in quest of something. A book to write, a picture to paint, a song to sing."*
> —*Henrietta Stein, resident*

On this early February morning, Henrietta Stein is sitting in her usual place at the dining table next to Lillian Garr. Partially blind, Lily is having trouble lifting her food from the tray to her mouth. The tray is too far away. Henrietta takes note of this and leans over to help. "Are you alright, honey?" she asks as she adjusts the tray within Lily's reach. Then, all hell breaks loose:

CARMA: That's NOT yours!
HENRIETTA: (quietly) I was trying to help her.
CARMA: I know, but don't touch her food.
ARNELLA: (sharply) Carma, I don't want her (Hennie) at the end of the table.
HENRIETTA: You better watch your tongue.
GLENDA: Well, you no longer touch her food.

The staff begin to move Henrietta's chair. "No-o-o-o-o-o," Henrietta screams. "Ohhhhh … You're hurting me. You're hurting me."

ARNELLA: Well, I'm sorry.
HENRIETTA: What are you DO-ing?
ARNELLA: You are not supposed to dig into other people's food.
HENRIETTA: What are you talking about? (looking up with disbelief)
GLENDA: You know …
HENRIETTA: No, this is my place.

ARNELLA: You have to move, Henrietta, because you can't stay out of that lady's tray.

HENRIETTA: (incredulously) What?!

ARNELLA: Get out of her tray.

HENRIETTA: Get out of whose tray? I wanted to show something to her, do something for her.

ARNELLA: You did …? (said in a condescending manner)

HENRIETTA: Yes, I did. Now leave me alone or I'll have you arrested. (Some residents laugh).

GLENDA: That's funny, isn't it Ruby?

HENRIETTA: Leave me alone. I'll call the police.

ARNELLA: No, Henrietta, you sit back over there.

HENRIETTA: Well, goddam it, YOU sit on the floor. (Resident Joan Bradford is watching and says, "Isn't that something?")

GLENDA: Yeh, she's got a bad mouth … a bad mouth.

ARNELLA: The one and only (speaking of Henrietta).

HENRIETTA: You took my chair from me.

CARMA: Well, you have a chair behind you.

HENRIETTA: That was my chair …

ARNELLA: I don't want anybody sitting here but Henrietta so she won't mess with anyone else's food.

HENRIETTA: You're a goddam nut. You have no right to take my chair from me. That's my chair.

CARMA: No, it's not Henrietta.

HENRIETTA: SHUT UP! (With that, resident Carrie Mae looks over at Henrietta and says, "Shut up.")

HENRIETTA: (Looking at Rita) SHUT up. You WILL shut up.

GLENDA: If you're going to talk like that we're going to have to send you away from here.

HENRIETTA: We'll have to get YOU away from here, Black bitch.

GLENDA: No, you're the trouble-maker.

HENRIETTA: You don't belong here.

GLENDA: Where do YOU belong?

HENRIETTA: I worked on drives to bring this place into realization …

GLENDA: We don't want to hear about that. We don't want to hear about that …

HENRIETTA: You don't want to hear about that. You're JEALOUS.

GLENDA: I don't have a thing to be jealous about. (With that, CNA Glenda moves away and Henrietta resumes her eating).

LPN Marita Martin is clear about Henrietta Stein:

> There's one resident who tries us. There's a hole. We're going to try to find and solve it. We all have different ideas except the one idea. We don't like

> being called out of our name. Nobody likes to be called black bitch, spick. So the girls are pretty excited about it. I told them to be patient with Henrietta. She is elderly. We have to keep her dignity and our respect for her intact.

Marita talks about staff being called a bunch of Kogies:

> When we want Hennie to change her dress we try to get her out of the outfit. She screams, "leave me alone." We are just asking her to change a dress because it is soiled. She says, "Get away from me." Then she calls us Kogies (Nigerians) and other things. Sometimes I think it's humorous. I really do, the way she comes off to us is like she's superior—*she's* superior.

Henrietta and the staff are entangled in a relationship ranging from acrimony, to standoffs, to explosions of feeling on both sides, to rare moments of fragile connection. Mis-communication devolving into anti-communication occurs often as the staff assume her guilty of misbehavior based on prior experience.

One of Nine Children

Henrietta Stein grew up in a small town, the seventh of nine children, and came to the city after high school to work for a small real estate company "keeping books." Speaking enthusiastically about "working with numbers," Henrietta was an accountant until her retirement at age sixty-five. She never married:

> My mother cried because all of her daughters remained single. There was a very nice young man who was after me. I was a bookkeeper and accountant. I was making good money and my sister and I were paying for our home. You pay for principle, interest and insurance, a new roof and new radiator. It uses your money up. The men in our family didn't pay for *anything*.

In the 1920s and 1930s, Henrietta was self-sufficient and ahead of her time in the pursuit of a career. She remains very proud of her work, her music lessons with a well-known teacher, her brother, a physician, and a sister, a bookkeeper who was "very dear" to her. A source of great satisfaction for Henrietta is having outlived all of her siblings. One morning as we sit in the sitting room, I ask about her sister Rachel:

ANNE: Your sister Rachel would be over one-hundred years of age now since you're ninety-four.

HENRIETTA: Is that how old I am?

ANNE: That's how old you are. (Henrietta looks up, grins, lifts her eyebrows, and wiggles her nose as though to usher in an important statement.)

HENRIETTA: Rachel was a good-looking lady.

ANNE: (in a playful tone) How would you describe yourself at that time?

HENRIETTA: I was a cutie (said with coyness and we laugh). I could have gotten married to a real nice boy but stepped aside helping to pay for the house. Tra la, la, la la la la (she begins to sing) I wish I could go away. That was a sad time. I could have married a very fine young man.

ANNE: So this young man wouldn't wait until you paid it off?

HENRIETTA: Which young man are you talking about?

ANNE: The one you told me about. Oh, you had several, huh? Now the truth comes Out. Maybe there were several (kidding tone).

HENRIETTA: (giggling) Yeh, there were.

Henrietta has a thick head of hair that resembles alabaster in its pure white color and smooth texture. A single wave caresses her right cheek. "Hey, I like your hair," I say. You had it cut and it looks good. "Yeh, Yeh," Hennie says. "They (the CNAs) did whatever they damn well pleased with it. They cut and cut and cut."

Henrietta Stein is a woman of "high intelligence," as some staff say, feistiness, and pride. She has been on the Pavilion for five years, having come from her private home to the independent living apartments at Starrmount. While an apartment resident, Henrietta became "disruptive," was reported to administration, and a place was found for her in the Alzheimer's Pavilion.[1]

Racism: Finding the Words to Say It

On a late Friday afternoon I talk with CNA Arnella about her work on the Pavilion and relationships with residents:

ARNELLA: Well, I think the attitudes down here are positive but there's one resident who tries us.

ANNE: Who is that?

ARNELLA: Henrietta. (laughs) Henrietta is ... (long pause) Let me see how can I put this. Very outspoken and she can say some very hurtful things.

ANNE: Like?

ARNELLA: (hesitating) She's very racial. She uses colors like "you black ——" (Arnella gestures with her index finger and makes lines in the air as a substitute for saying a word she wants to avoid). That is just how she is. Like for instance I saw one of the residents accidentally hit her chair. By the time she turned around that person was gone and someone else was standing over there by the chair and she hit them. I asked her why she did that and she said because they hit her. And I said, "No, they didn't." She started tearing into me (laughs).

ANNE: With racial statements?

ARNELLA: Uh huh. Black bitch. N——. This happens every day around mealtime. It's like she gets agitated for some reason. For one thing she likes to have her tray first. But we can't dig through all the trays to get hers. For some residents we have to do this because they'll leave if we don't. With her, she's not going to leave. She's going to sit up there and go on and on about her tray and coffee (laughter).

ANNE: Has the group gotten together to do anything about this?

ARNELLA: I think everybody deals with this on their own. I mean we don't deny her care but sometimes, I try to stay away from her. I try to leave her alone if she's not in the best of moods.

Arnella's initial hesitation to "name" Henrietta's racism gives way as we talk but she reveals as little as she can about how she defines Henrietta's racist behavior toward the staff. At first, she is reluctant to give words to what Henrietta says to the African-American CNAs but relents a bit when she says, "Let me see how I can put this," an indication she must couch her comments in acceptable language and not *name* Henrietta's statements for what they are, racist. Arnella does not initiate claims of racism but leaves it to others to name the offensive behavior, which may give her permission to say what is the case, after which she elaborates with more detail.

Racism on the Pavilion is complicated. Henrietta flaunts her racism and classism and makes sure to point out that there are "too many Schwartz, the German word for Blacks," on the Pavilion. In contrast, some residents display what can be called a "veiled racism." Boris Randolph expresses veiled racism when he murmurs to me one day when figuring out where to sit at the dining table, "Well she's Black, ah, but … I guess I can sit over there by her anyway, maybe." Resident Harriet French, strolls by me, swaying back and forth, and whispers in a negative tone, "You know that dark person, that dark-er person over there" (pointing to Justine), "She really thinks she's something. Yes, she sure does."

Staff's relationship with Henrietta Stein reveals the contradiction between how they live in the midst of acts of racism and classism and yet deny their existence or minimize their impact. When defining the meaning of the Pavilion as a refuge, Marita Martin speaks passionately,

> It feels like an island sometimes, yeh, and I hate to get off this island sometimes … hate to go out that door into the larger world (said with much feeling and some tearing). I'm serious, into the outside world. Because, you know here I'm safe. We don't see prejudice. We don't see no bigotry. We don't see hate between people. We see arguments, but we don't see hate. We see a lot of love some days. We are a unit, not as in ward or facility but a unit, as in family.

Other than Justine, who never refers to Henrietta in our discussions, Marita, Arnella, Carma Lee and Chevelle, at first, avoid explicit examples and name Henrietta's behavior as "being very trying," "Henrietta says things that are hurtful," and "She doesn't say very nice things," all euphemisms. CNA Glenda, however, does not hesitate to be candid in her description of Henrietta. With eagerness, she blurts out, "Henrietta Stein is just a snotty person, an old snotty person. Mean and real dirty, real dirty person." With palpable disdain in the telling, Glenda provides details:

> Hennie will say, "Oh, you don't know what you're talking about. I helped build this place. You're black and you don't know anything. You goddam n——." She says this everyday. She's calling somebody a spick. There was another charge nurse down here and I must have said something and Hennie called me a n——. The nurse said, "Oh Hen. You don't talk like that now. I won't have you talking like this." Hennie says, "Oh, you're just a n—— lover." The first time it happened I was pretty upset. I just walked away. Now, it doesn't bother me because it happens so much. But it bothers me because she *knows* what she's doing. Now, I might laugh at her. She says, "I graduated with honors and you don't know anything." She's set in her ways and won't change. She's different than the other residents. She's more alert and knows more.

Glenda's reactions to the racist comments reveal a conflict and an important distinction. On the one hand, the *words* themselves, while stinging, no longer "bother" her because of their frequency; racist comments may lose the power of their thrust through habituation. On the other hand, the *intention* behind the comments does bother Glenda because she views Henrietta as aware (conscious) of what she says and does. Most of the time, as a means of coping, Marita and the CNAs attribute residents' abusive behavior and language to the disease; however, they cannot do the same with Henrietta because they do not consider her to be a "true Alzheimer's." Some CNAs attribute her abusive language to cultural upbringing, while others "try to ignore it." What is unknown is the deeper impact of continual racial slurs that tread on the CNAs' most fundamental identity, their racial identity, by calling them "out of their name."

CNA Chevelle indicates how her reactions toward Henrietta have changed over time:

> Henrietta knows she has the upper hand. So you can't just confront her. I just try and ignore it. At first, I was angry and I asked her where did she learn such language, like black bitch. I shouldn't have said anything. I said, "You're always saying you're a Jewish lady and ladies don't talk like that." She just came back at me more.

Chevelle appeals to Henrietta's moral stance as a "Jewish lady." She uses "inquiry" first and then admonishment to deal with Hennie's racist remarks. In the end, Chevelle "tries to ignore it," which intimates an ongoing discipline of sorts which weighs on the CNAs but may be assuaged by their relationship with other residents.

CNA Carma "thinks out loud" about Henrietta's behavior and comes to a conclusion:

> She did not go to college but did graduate from high school with honors and that's why she uses some of the words that she does. I don't know if she realizes it or not. (pause) Well, she does realize it. She belittles other people.

Carma Lee employs a euphemism, "belittles," for racism. Even when she equivocates regarding intentionality as she considers whether Henrietta "realizes" she is belittling others (e.g. "I don't know if she realizes it or not. Well, she does realize it.") Carma adds an additional layer of avoidance in "naming" Henrietta's behavior by leaving it to the very end of her statement. Carma Lee holds contradictory feelings about Henrietta based on her philosophy of care work:

> It means a lot. It might not mean a lot to other people. It means a lot of caring, giving. Don't have any room for color. There's no color. There shouldn't be anyway. Seeing human beings as they really are, regardless of how much money they have, how rich they were at one time or how prominent they were at one time. Even when that is all taken away they are still a human being.

Carma states, "There's no color. Don't have any room for color." In principle, Carma allows for the possibility of color (prejudice or racism) on the Pavilion with an amendment to her preceding statement, "There *shouldn't* be (color) anyway."

The minimizing of talk about racism/classism in contrast to the maximizing of talk about the collective construction of their different care work in the Pavilion is noteworthy. Several possible reasons come to mind. First, the staff may be reticent to reveal an issue with negative valence for which they do not have a solution. Second, CNAs construct another "reality" and just "ignore it." Third, they may not want to expose the "hole" to me because it may reflect negatively on their identity and cast aspersions on the rest of their work. Fourth, they may fear retribution associated with what they perceive to be Henrietta's social position within the larger institution and community. "I don't know how the staff take it (racial slurs)," RN Elaine Pressley says. Carma Lee notes, "I guess that we all have our own way of dealing with it." There is an avoidance of a discussion *among* the staff about the intractable problem of blatant racism.

Henrietta as "Trouble"

It is mid-morning when Henrietta ambles up while I am chatting with Marita and says "hi." She turns to Marita and the following takes place:

> HENRIETTA: (to Marita) Honey, will you please get me some coffee with milk and sugar?

MARITA: (not looking up from her work, in a corrective tone) Now, Henrietta you know what I have told you and we are going to get into an AR-GU-ment.

HENRIETTA: (very calmly) There's no argument.

MARITA: (emphatically) No! you can't have it. (Things are starting to heat up and one can feel the intensity from Marita but not from Hennie)

HENRIETTA: Why must it be like this? Why do you have to speak like this? (More back and forth occurs).

MARITA: (commanding tone) Will you please leave?

HENRIETTA: Why? (The delicate tide turns. Where once the exchange had a chance to have created a different dialogue just a second before with Henrietta's question there is an abrupt halt. With her appeal having been denied, Hennie now goes on the offensive).

HENRIETTA: YOU leave. I pay your salary. I pay YOU.

Henrietta stands in place continuing to look at Marita. Marita says nothing and stonewalls until Henrietta leaves. "This is the umpteenth time that Henrietta pulls this and she *knows* she cannot have coffee, physician's orders. The way to handle this is to ignore her," Marita comments. Before ignoring, however, Marita sets up a situation, interactionally, from which she cannot return.

There is a sub-text underlying the CNAs' interaction with Henrietta which constructs and anticipates Henrietta as 'trouble.'[2] While the staff may deal with racism *individually*, the CNAs, as a *group*, have constructed responses to Henrietta Stein's customary ways of acting and speaking to the staff. The relationship between Henrietta and the staff has not improved but become an entrenched form of interaction that constructs each as the enemy of the other where all parties are on guard. A contest of wills is ever-present. To emphasize its rarity, Marita highlights what she characterizes as "only two days of getting along with Henrietta for as long as I can remember":

> One particular morning Hennie was so well behaved. She loved all of us including the Black girls. I'm thinking maybe it's because she has her own toilet paper. They issued two rolls of toilet paper to her. Nobody can touch these rolls. We started giving her Postum but we had to quit because she kept getting diarrhea severe. She had her Caffeine. She was happy. The girls tried to please her tremendously that day. We had two good days. Then all of a sudden she walked through the back of the desk (nurse's alcove) and we have these notes up there 'for staff only.' She persisted she was going to take a short cut. Nobody else takes a short cut. So, that day everything ended.

When Henrietta Stein first came to the Pavilion, her adjustment was impeded by what Marita Martin describes as "desertion" by the members of the synagogue who pushed to have her admitted:

MARITA: Henrietta was living at the Plaza in her own little room. What happened was that she wasn't keeping it the way she should. She was neglecting her hygiene. She would put something on the stove and forget it. So they saw dementia coming on and transferred her here.

ANNE: Does she know why she's here?

MARITA: I don't think so and even if she does she has probably just flat out blocked it out. One of the synagogues had pressured us, "You have to take her." For the first two weeks they came to see her every day. Then all of a sudden they cut her off. That's what angers me. She wanted to go to that congregation. But they won't come and pick her up and then it fell on us to make excuses which I thought was unfair to her. Even if they would come once a month I would be ecstatic about it. It's not even that anymore. We've called and they say, "well if we can find someone to go out there." I don't understand. Surely there's someone who could give her ten to fifteen minutes of their time to come and visit. We had a problem getting a Jewish calendar for her. Why? They said they would send it in the mail. We are still waiting for it. This was last year. Their attention lasted a month.

ANNE: Did she enjoy their visits?

MARITA: Oh yeh, she would be so excited. She gets excited about anything if it's centered around her. But then aren't we all? We all get excited if we get a call. I think that was very cruel of them to cut her off.

ANNE: What happened when she first came in and saw the Pavilion?

MARITA: Let me tell you what happened. She came to us and she told us that "Geriatric means for sick people." I said, "Oh, no that means elderly." She would just look at me and say, "I don't know why I'm here." Time went on … and she stayed.

From Marita's point of view the staff have tried every strategy they know to "make Henrietta happy" and to "make themselves happy in working with her." She explains:

> But, same ol' Henrietta. We were just waiting for the lid to blow off because I knew she was going to complain about something. She doesn't have friends and a family that visits her … she had a cousin who came over and I just couldn't believe it. But with Henrietta's mannerisms I wouldn't want to be her friend. She doesn't appreciate anything. You can go out of your way for her and she doesn't appreciate it. She feels you owe it to her.

Throughout this conversation one can detect anger in Marita's voice that gives way to weariness. Most residents have degrees of social appropriateness that serve as a regulator of behavior but Henrietta splinters race and class boundaries head on. "I pay your salaries. You wouldn't have a job if it weren't for me," she proclaims.

Constructing Interaction

One afternoon just before leaving for the day, Marita Martin wants to talk with me about a recent "incident" with Henrietta Stein when she volunteered to take Hennie to the eye doctor:

> The problem mainly concerned money. When we got there Henrietta stood up in the waiting room and says, "I don't have the money to pay for eye glasses." You know how she does her little gesture (Henrietta standing with her chest puffed up and her hands raised on either side of her chest with her fingers coming forward in a gesture as if she is putting her hands through an imaginary pair of suspenders and thrusting them forward). I tell her I will take care of it. When we get back from the eye doctor the taxi cab stops in front of the front entrance at Starrmount. Hennie says, "I'm not getting out here. I live over there" (pointing to the independent apartments). I said, "But now you live over HERE". So, I finally had to get a guy from engineering to go out there and tell her this is where she lives.

Henrietta is well aware that she no longer lives in the apartments but uses this occasion to stand her ground, according to Marita. Of all the staff, interaction and the consequences are most volatile between Marita and Henrietta. Marita adds,

> There is no one she gets along with well. I'll go out of my way to do special things for her cause I feel the way I do. Because sometimes I don't think I'm fair with her. I don't know if you've ever disliked someone to the point where when they even say hello to you it kinda grabs ya. I, we clash.

As I observed interaction over the course of a year and a half on the Pavilion several patterns emerged between Henrietta Stein and the staff, all of which led to non-communication between the two.

Henrietta's Strategies

> It's around 8:15 am on a rainy Friday. As I enter the Pavilion I hear raucous exchanges coming from the vicinity of Henrietta's room. I can make out Hennie's scream, "Room 9, Room 9, severe diarrhea." CNAs Arnella and Chevelle are running toward the room to help Hennie and keep her from dragging the waste along the hallway. She has eaten the forbidden Postum cereal and all are dealing with the results. In this case, Henrietta lays in bed waiting for the CNAs. Later, Marita comments to me: "She can help herself. You know, for showing the independence she has, she doesn't. So we go in there. The girls have to give her a bath. She doesn't want a bath because it's

not her bath day and she knows this. Finding out about the Postum, I hated it, I just hated it."

A dominant strategy Henrietta uses in interaction with the CNAs and Marita is assuming privilege. This privilege is manifested in her racist remarks and in claims of what the CNAs say is "superiority" based on her former social position in the community. Henrietta's taking cereal from the nurse's alcove angers Marita for two reasons. First, from Marita's perspective, Henrietta "knows better" and yet defies the sign on the wall, "staff only." She assumes she is privileged and can do what others are denied. From the CNA's perspective, such actions confirm Henrietta as trouble over and over again. Second, eating the Postum cereal will cause Henrietta to have "dreaded" diarrhea, which creates temporary mayhem on the Pavilion and unnecessary work for the staff.

According to the CNAs, Henrietta's assumption of privilege can be seen in mundane activities. One day, I notice Henrietta looking around the family room to see if anyone is watching. She picks up something from the sitting area, stashes it under her arm as if to hide it, and makes a beeline for her room. Later in the day, Marita tells me that "Henrietta's grumpy when she wakes up 'Where's my paper?'" she says. "You know how she does. So we give it to her and she goes back to her room and hides it under her pillow. We know her hiding places. She comes back, ta-DA, ta-DA, ta-DA, ta-DA (singing). You know how she does those cute little gestures" (said with a hint of sarcasm). Henrietta's behavior cannot be separated from the history of the troubled relationship with staff, her "name calling," and the "intentionality" attributed to her by the staff.

Henrietta uses a second strategy of attempting to *appeal* to staff or ask if she can be of assistance. One morning after breakfast Henrietta sits near the TV in her usual chair, avidly watching a program. Marita comes over to the sitting room to adjust the TV:

Henrietta asks Marita, "Can I do anything for you?" (from her tone of voice Henrietta is asking if she can be of help, not to interfere or cause problems. It is possible Hennie's approach stemmed from the moments of collective singing a few minutes earlier at the table). Marita responds (curtly) "No!" (She does not make eye contact with Hennie). What could have been a pivotal moment of communication passes. Soon Henrietta (now loudly responding "in kind") "You're in my way, you're in my way" (nasty tone). Marita continues to stand in front of the TV. CNA Diane comes over to give Marita the key to the television. CNA Diane says in a mocking way, "Marita, did you hear that you are in Henrietta's way?" They both smile, knowingly. The exchange becomes a power struggle, an unequal one at that. What begins as an appeal ends with reactivity from both Henrietta and Marita. Any possibility of continuing the interactional process toward shared meaning is defeated. On the one hand, Henrietta's overture to Marita may be interpreted as a resident's desire to reclaim some measure of self-determination and control. On the other hand, from the staff's perspective, it provides confirmation of Henrietta as "trouble."

Staff Strategies

Several residents remain at the dining table after lunch as I sit and talk with Henrietta. She is intent on showing me and resident Ruby Klein what Matzo bread (a brittle, flat piece of unleavened bread eaten at Passover) looks like. She asks CNA Glenda if she can find some more Matzo. Glenda tells her there isn't any more. Henrietta inquires if there is any in the refrigerator and would Glenda look for it because she wants to show someone what it looks like. Glenda says, "Uh HUH." Her facial expression, raised eyebrows, and tone of voice indicate she doubts Henrietta's motives and assumes she is up to her old tricks. Several times in a nice manner, Henrietta asks the same question. Finally, Glenda gives in and gets some Matzo from the refrigerator. Henrietta hands us each a jellied piece after which she asks if she can have some hot tea. A substitute aide for the day calls to Henrietta, "You want some, I'll get it Hennie." "Thank you dear," Henrietta says, and calls to the cleaning man who just arrived. "Here comes that hard-working guy," she says. "That's right. How you doin', Miss Henrietta," he says with a smile. The contrast and approach in interaction is striking. In contrast to the exchange between Glenda and Hennie, dialogue with the substitute aide and cleaning man advantages Henrietta. She is seen, publicly, as "not trouble" having accomplished a satisfactory exchange in interaction.

With a set of assumptions in place about who Hennie is and what she will do, the CNAs and Marita Martin miss opportunities to take their exchange toward shared meaning. In this chapter's opening scene, Hennie is "accused" of something she did not do, namely, taking food from resident Lily's plate. At first, Henrietta defends herself and explains what she is doing to assist Lily who is almost blind. From the point at which the CNAs move Hennie's chair with her in it, the interaction escalates into accusations, misinterpretations, and the CNAs' faulty constructions of what happened. Henrietta becomes enraged and peppers her responses with racist comments confirming the staff's perspective. From the *first* point of interaction, the CNAs act on their assumption that Henrietta is up to no good and are unwilling or unable to change their view even when Hennie tries to explain herself.

A second interactional approach CNAs use with Henrietta is what I call mocking or having a sarcastic commentary on her interactions: During the late morning, residents are listening to music. Resident Boots (Verna) is clapping and singing along with the music. Henrietta attempts to assert control over the situation and announces, "Be still." Arnella, who is standing nearby catches Henrietta's comment and turns to Marita and the CNAs to say (in a mocking tone), "Henrietta says to be still." Another example involves Marita relating a story to the other aides about a woman in a fast food store who was very demanding and nasty and she then says, "Who does that remind you of?" Arnella says, "Hennnnnn-rietta." The practice of keeping alive the perspective of Henrietta as trouble is accomplished through re-telling the event later in the day to RN Elaine Pressley.

The staff's habituation and exhaustion in relating to Henrietta Stein have solidified and hardened into a mode of reaction. The co-construction of trouble is accomplished by Hennie in the course of the interaction which confirms the label. The staff have become used to responding in a manner the opposite of communication which involves aligning oneself with the other again and again to reach shared meaning and taking the attitude of the other as your own.

Spontaneous Connections

It's lunchtime on the Pavilion. The cleaning man and another aide are in the corridor near the door and Henrietta is at the table. Glenda walks by quickly and gets her back support entangled on the chair and it stops her with her right leg dangling in mid-air. The other aides notice Henrietta laughing. Glenda looks over at Henrietta in a good-natured way and says: "What you laughin' at Henrietta?" The cleaning man says, "That was funny wasn't it Henrietta?" They all laugh and then Henrietta plays it down and controls her laughter but directly after, she sings in a carefree manner.

At this moment there is human sharing in laughter regardless of race and class. Other examples involve spontaneous dancing and singing. Every once and while, Henrietta will dance a little jig. One day Arnella walks by and in a playful manner says, "You want to dance, do ya Henrietta." As she passes, Arnella wiggles her hips to join with Hennie's gyrations. Henrietta may start singing wherever she is at the moment, many times during or after lunch. Immediately, the CNAs, Marita, and some residents will join in the collective exuberance, sometimes with fragments of word and melody, sometimes with clarity of lyrics. These spontaneous bursts of creative energy offer a brief reprieve from the underlying conflict.

Ambivalence typifies some CNAs' feelings toward Henrietta Stein. Her level of alertness provides a "stimulus" for the staff provided it does not result in problematic behavior. In spite of Henrietta's treatment of them, several CNAs mention they have a "fascination with" or "attraction to" her intelligence. Classism, using class to declare privilege and superiority over others, as some of the staff think Henrietta does with them is one thing; however, CNAs can put a positive valence on exhibitions of class in that it gives them a glimpse into a world they would never have in the outside society. Strategies of the staff to ignore Henrietta's racist remarks can be interpreted as a means of erasure, to make the remarks impotent, so as not to experience what they experience in the outside world.[3]

In a final reflection on Henrietta Stein, Marita declares,

> We're not doing enough for her. But we're all falling into this category. We had a meeting and agreed that we do have holes there that we need to fix. We need to patch them up emotionally with her as far as support goes.

Whereas Henrietta Stein represents one kind of trouble on the Pavilion, families represent a different kind of collective challenge for the staff.

Notes

1 In the case of Henrietta, the independent living apartment dwellers (her community) reacted to her careless behavior and breaking of the rules. What may have been idiosyncratic behavior was labeled "mentally ill," deviant behavior; she was deemed unable to live without supervision. Societal reaction is a powerful social control mechanism with emotional and practical consequences. In Henrietta Stein's case, she was banished to the Alzheimer's Pavilion. For more on residual rule-breaking, see Thomas Scheff, *Being Mentally Ill: A Sociological Theory* (Piscataway, NJ: Aldine Transaction Publishers, 1999: 19).

2 See the classic article by Robert Emerson and Sheldon Messinger, "The Micro-Politics of Trouble," *Social Problems*, 25 (1977): 121–134; also see Jaber F. Gubrium and Margaretha Järvinen (eds), *Turning Troubles into Problems: Clientization in Human Services* (London: Routledge, 2014); and Jaber F. Gubrium, Tone Alm Andreassen, and Per Koren (eds), *Reimagining the Human Service Relationship* (New York: Columbia University Press, 2016).

3 For additional discussion on race, care work and relationships see: Celia Berdes and John M. Eckert, "Race Relations and Caregiving Relationships: A Qualitative Perspective From Residents and Aides in Three Nursing Homes," *Research on Aging* 23 (2001): 109–126; Lisa Dodson, Rebekah Zincavage, "It's Like a Family: Caring Labor, Exploitation, and Race in Nursing Homes," *Gender and Society* 21 (2007): 905–928; Sharon Harley. "Speaking Up: The Politics of Black Women's Labor History," in E. Higginbotham and Mary Romero (eds), *Women and Work: Exploring Race, Ethnicity, and Class* (Thousand Oaks, CA: Sage Publications, 1997: 28–51); and Evelyn Nakano Glenn, "Racial Ethnic Women's Labor: The Intersection of Race, Gender and Class Oppression," *Review of Radical Political Economics* 17 (1985): 86–108.

6

DEFENDING THE ETHIC OF CARE

Intrusions

On a snowy winter morning, as I make my way over to the sitting area, I am distracted by voices coming from outside the nurses' alcove. CNAs Justine, Arnella, and LPN Marita Martin are in a heated conversation. They are discussing the behavior of Don Jacobson whose wife was moved from the Pavilion to the non-ambulatory Alzheimer's unit six months ago. In spite of the move, every night when he comes to the unit, he brings his wife over to the Pavilion. Justine explains what she thinks is "Jacobson taking over" in a place where he shouldn't be:

JUSTINE: I said to him, "ok, but I don't want this every evening because the evenings I am here I'm going to be watching you."

MARITA: What was he doing this time?

JUSTINE: He's done exactly what he's wanted to. Pushes residents around. Talks mean to them and oh, I just can't stand it. You know, I liked him at first and then I would follow him and this made him mad. Well, he knows somebody on the Board. I've told him: "I don't care who you are or who you know but they have families that love them just like you love your wife and I don't think that they would take too kindly to the abuse that you are giving. I'm going to be watching you." Remember that, Arnella?

ARNELLA: Yes.

JUSTINE: I made him mad. But I told him, "your wife is going to live longer than you anyway because you're so mean to the residents here." It seems like they are trying to abuse them or something. I don't know. That makes me angry. He comes over here, turns on the TV to what he wants and he's verbally abusive to the residents. Oh, he has even grabbed and twisted

> and hit. I've reported it but Greenberg's not doing a thing about it. Like I've told the CEO, I said, "I don't care if I'd lose my job, but I'll lose it by protecting them not because I'm hurting them."

I witness Don Jacobson's behavior one late afternoon as he arrives in the family room. He plops on one end of the couch where I am sitting, stretches his legs out, and pulls his wife who is in a wheel chair alongside. Immediately, he screams at resident Mattie Gardner, "Stop digging in your pants. NOW. Did you hear me, stop it. DID you hear me?" Shaking his head in a disapproving manner when Mattie does not comply, he grabs her arm as she comes near him and yanks it out of her pants. Ralph Fraser, son of another resident sits between us on the sofa. Shaking his head, Don turns to Ralph and says, "You know they all have some kind of story." Across the room, Henrietta Stein is watching TV and Ralph Fraser yells to her, "Hey Hennie, what kind of work did YOU do?" Henrietta turns and looks in his direction without answering. Again, Don yells, "Did you hear me, Hennie?" With that, Henrietta stands up, turns her back to him, and marches out of the sitting room, head held high.

These incidents pose an order of threats which CNAs define as "abuse" of residents. For staff, all actions matter and have consequences. The problematic treatment of residents can be consequential in two ways. First, it can diminish the Pavilion ethic of respect for the personhood of residents. Second, it can exacerbate resident agitation, which may snowball to other residents, cause disruption of the prevailing order, and create more work for CNAs. While some might argue that Justine's approach is not the best method, nonetheless, she is defending an ethic through resident advocacy.

Carma Lee speaks to how a CNA's autonomy may be threatened when family is on the Pavilion:

> You never know who's watching you. I found that out by experience. Make sure you cover yourself particularly on falls and be detailed about what happened. I feel a pair of eyes when the family members are here both for my residents and about what family says about the whole unit. If they think you are mistreating a resident then they are going to say, "What goes on with my family member?" Be on your guard.

The Pavilion is both a refuge and a site of struggle where CNAs protect their autonomy and defend their ethic of care[1] in relation to families. Charge nurse, Marita and her staff maintain the boundaries of the Pavilion through a normative structure that dictates how people should act and treat each other while on the Pavilion. This structure, which I term an ethic of care, is composed of a set of behavioral expectations best expressed as a recognition of respect for residents and staff and for the skills and knowledge of the CNAs. Justine's unequivocal pronouncement to the substitute aide, "... we don't talk to our residents the way you just did. No sir-ee. We, ah, do things just a LIT…tle differently down here" underscores the valence connected with those "little" differences.

On Display: Resident-as-Object

CNA Chevelle, CNA Glenda and I discuss resident behavior during lunch one day in proximity to a daughter and her mother who are viewing the residents. The daughter says, "I saw 'one' (a resident) shit in her pants. It's funny in one way and it's not. But I guess you have to have something to keep up your spirits." Chevelle and Carma are aware of the conversation as am I. Mother and daughter continue to gaze at residents moving in various regions of the room and the daughter comments on the groupings:

> They are just back and forth all the time. It seems funny to sit and look at 'em. This one (pointing to the resident) has decided to make bloomers out of hers and has rolled up her pants (both mother and daughter are laughing out loud). She's wearing shorts. I think half of them are reliving their childhood, really.

As we walk away from the scene, CNA Glenda whispers, "I've seen this before and it still makes me mad." Both Glenda and Diane have come to recognize this behavior as one of the ways a family member may act out the perspective, "my mother or father is not like these other people." At the same time, CNAs experience it as an intrusion on their ethic of respect as a behavioral principle. The need for family members to distance their loved one from the collective "other" may take different forms. Paulina Creed's daughter tells me that the way she holds on to "who my Mother really is" is to take her out of the Pavilion and visit in the upstairs main lobby of Starrmount Geriatric. By taking Paulina off the Pavilion, she also negates the possibility of connecting with the staff. As well, from time to time, friends accompany the family or come on their own to visit particular residents. CNAs note that they will stare at the resident as if the resident were an object. The "staring phenomenon" is described by Carma Lee:

> People who accompany family. One of several cases is a woman who had known Marge Jacobs back when Marge was well known in the city. She was staring at her like she was on display or something. She just watched her the whole time and I thought it was so rude even though Marge didn't realize what the woman was doing, but *we* did.

Another example of objectifying a resident involves a daughter not wanting other residents to touch her mother. When the daughter comes to visit, she takes her to another part of the room to avoid the other residents' behavior. CNA Justine contends that it is very difficult to get the daughter to see that her mother "does those very things" about which the daughter is complaining. Justine takes a confrontational approach and tells the daughter, "I hope you don't treat your mother like you are treating them." With a different approach, Arnella elaborates on how she deals with resident objectification through avoidance:

> Residents like to touch people. They're not going to hurt you. The children act a little better than the adults do. They'll let them hug them and they'll talk to them. But some of the adults they will run from them like something's wrong—like they're contagious—it's very, very annoying. When I see that a visitor has come in and one of the residents goes up to talk to them and their loved one, I will go up and tell them, "Come on, come with me," because I don't like anybody to be abusive to them whether its physically or verbally. I have seen times when people will just take their hands and just kind of push them away. I don't like that, not one bit.

Arnella grimaces when she gestures with her hands to demonstrate how adults "will take their hands and just push them (the residents) away." Such action is "very, very annoying" to her and she provides active protection from potential physical or verbal abuse. The affront has been felt and registered with Arnella. She is affected even though it is unknown if or how the intended recipient, the resident, experienced the offense. She foresees the possibility of uncontrollable behavior that may agitate the other residents and circumvents it. From another perspective, Arnella's taking on the shame and the act of telling me allows the demeaning behavior to be registered in another human being. From time to time, CNAs experience what Bogdin and Taylor[2] say is a "contempt toward outsiders who reveal by their remarks, tone of voice, or actions that they are uncomfortable in the presence of the disabled person or find the relationship odd." The CNAs, however, differ from the able and disabled persons in the Bogdan and Taylor study, with the latter both sharing contempt for outsiders. The CNAs cannot be clear on what feelings residents might have toward outsiders whom the CNAs see as contemptible in their disrespect and abuse of residents.

As seasoned watchers of verbal and non-verbal behavior, Carma Lee, her teammates, and Marita are acutely aware of the actions and language that outsiders (a number of families and others) use in relating to residents. I can attest to the CNAs' skill set in this area. During an interview with CNA Justine eight months after I came to the Alzheimer's Pavilion, I asked her about the staff's reaction to my being on the Pavilion. Without missing a beat and with a wry smile on her face, she said, "We wanted to see how you were going to treat the residents." I was on trial; my probationary period ended when one of the CNAs failed to notice me as she passed by. When I commented on her lapse, she immediately laughed and said, "My gosh, Anne, you've become so much a part of the unit, I didn't even notice you sitting there."

In their role as care workers, Arnella emphasizes that "we are there for all residents" regardless of their relationship with family members. At a minimum, they have a perfunctory role with families as Marita explains: "Just some families have involved themselves with us. You know, I like to keep in touch with them and let them know what's going on." In their struggles with families, staff employ a changing repertoire of tactics such as direct confrontation, being "on guard," avoidance, and at times, entering into a fragile connection (although many times ephemeral) with family members. Overall, CNAs have a churning emotional mix of dislike and regard for families depending on how they treat their loved one and other residents and how they treat the CNAs.

Ambivalence and Threats to Autonomy

As he slowly descends the stairs in front of Starrmount Geriatric Center and walks across the parking lot, his crouched upper body bears the weight of an intractable burden of loss. Stanley Braun will not let a day go by without visiting his wife, Leah. All the days I was on the Pavilion, I watched him leave with a heavy heart. He carries within him what he says is a "living sadness," the one constant emotional connection with Leah.

Theirs' had been a vibrant life. She was a vigorous and stylish woman who loved to dance. During my interview with Mr. Braun in his home, he brings out a collection of photographs of Leah through the years. As we turn the pages of the album, he talking and lingering on this or that image, I taking in what seemed more like the resurrection of a life than a remembrance, my eyes came to rest on her portrait over the fireplace. Noticing that I am staring at the beautiful rendering of his wife, Mr. Braun murmurs, "So alive." Then, as though a fire has turned to ashes right before his eyes, his expression becomes leaden as he tells me about the first time he took her to day care at the Alzheimer's Pavilion. "She would ask, 'Why are you doing this to me?' I just couldn't do it anymore and took her home. But, finally I had to admit her."

Stanley Braun is one of those spouses with whom most CNAs have an ambivalent relationship. CNA Justine articulates one of the problems that interferes with the staff's commitment to teamwork, that is, asking for one CNA all the time and criticizing others:

> What bothers us about him is the fact that, don't single one of us out. He's gotten so that he asks for me. Because I as well as Arnella as well as Carma Lee all take care of his wife. There's no one person that is better than the other. Not as far as we are concerned, because we all are family here. We are together and we do teamwork down here. Don't single me out because I am not always here. So don't pat me on the back and turn around and snap at my co-workers because we all do the same thing.

Justine tells me that she has learned to "disappear" when Mr. Braun comes. One can appreciate Justine's allegiance to teamwork, to share the burden of Mr. Braun so she does not have to shoulder his needs by herself. She opts for self-protection.

The Brauns' daughter interrupts the CNAs' care work with her constant complaints. CNAs make special preparations when she comes. A staff member relates,

> Leah has a couple of daughters. One of them is out of town and has a very difficult time with her mother being here. They would tell us when she's coming so we could make sure Leah takes a nap and have everything kinda special when the daughter comes. Have the mother looking special because the daughter is having so much difficulty.

The impetus for making unusual preparations stems from both a concern for Mr. Braun and Leah as well as a deterrent to the daughter's complaining. I ask Arnella how the daughter is expressing her difficulty:

> She cries and complains about her care and her looks. She thinks she should look like she used to. Of course nothing is ever good enough for your mother. If Leah drops something on her clothes when they were feeding her or something like that, the daughter looks at the clothes and the hair. We usually try to get her in the beauty shop and stay there with her and hold her steady if we can without being too forceful if she doesn't like it. Sometimes, I'll roll her hair and she'll walk around with the rollers which she does fine with but she doesn't like to sit.

The need of family members, such as the Braun's daughter, to have her mother "look like she used to," is an intrusion on the CNA's practice of accepting and nurturing the resident's "new self" as a member of the Pavilion. The staff feel ambivalent toward Mr. Braun in that they react negatively to his everyday intrusions; at the same time they try to understand and help a man who is angry and forlorn.

From another perspective, what the staff experience as intrusive, troublesome family behavior may be understood on a deeper level as a change of Leah Braun's "place" in the family as a result of Alzheimer's disease. Erving Goffman provides a conceptual framework on the importance of one's "place" in the family as a social organization that provides insight into families such as the Brauns. In "The Insanity of Place," Goffman[3] addresses the connection of one's place with the internal functioning of the family (emphases are the author's):

> There is the obligation of each member to care and protect the others, insofar as they are in need of this help and a member is able to provide it. There is a normatively established allocation of respect, affection and moral support. Some common values and social ways of doing things will be

> maintained. A crisscross of personal relationships will be sustained. As a special feature of the family as a social organization, each member commits his own dealings and involvement to what he takes to be the personal interests and personal plight of each of the others. *In brief the activity of each member tends to express that he knows what his social place is in the family and that he is sticking to it.* The maintenance of the internal and external functioning of the family is so central that when family members think of the essential character, the perduring personality of any one of their numbers, it is usually his habitual patterns of support for family-organized activity and family relationships, his style of acceptance of this place in the family that they have in mind. Any marked change in his pattern of support will tend to be perceived as a marked change in his character. (Family) feel bewildered by the change in character and personality that has occurred.

Stanley Braun is a man who is bewildered and who resides in a living sadness due to changes in his wife, Leah, as a result of the assaults of Alzheimer's disease. In the context of Goffman's perspective, it can be argued that his wife's change in place from a woman who was "so alive" and loved to dance to what he calls "a lost soul" is not only a source of considerable personal grief for Mr. Braun, but also a loss of his wife's place in the functioning of the family. Leah's inability to maintain her part in what Goffman refers to as the "allocation of respect, affection and moral support"[4] within the internal functioning of the family becomes devastating. As well, the daughter's constant complaining and her desire to have her mother "look like she used to" may be prompted by a latent feeling of her mother not keeping her place in both the inward functioning and the outward impression of the family.

Intrusions on autonomy can come in the form of confrontations initiated by male spouses, and can arise unexpectedly, as in this example:

> Most residents are dozing at this hour of the morning right after breakfast. Several carts of resident clothing are in full view at the far end of the Pavilion where the CNAs appear to be discussing the sorting process. As the group disbands, Mr. Andrews, resident Patsy's husband and a daily visitor to the Pavilion, approaches Arnella. "That woman (pointing to Ruby Klein) has got my wife's clothes on," he says. "What's she doing wearing her clothes?" His voice rises steadily in volume. Arnella responds that she believes the clothes are Ruby's but, "I will certainly look into it right away. In fact, I will get Glenda who helped Ruby dress this morning to come over." In a huffy manner, Mr. Andrews declares, "I will certainly bring this up to Marita Martin when I see her." Glenda comes over and verifies that these are indeed Ruby's clothes. The husband continues to shout in an accusatory tone, "Those clothes look just like my wife's so they must be hers." Instead of denying again that the clothes belong to the wife, Arnella and Glenda try to de-intensify the situation by telling the husband that they will check

> later and if it turns out that they are his wife's they will be "returned immediately." At this point, Mr. Andrew's daughter, who has accompanied him and is sitting on the couch nearby, glances up and says, "Hey Dad, when they made that one outfit they didn't stop makin' them. Several people have those outfits." With a smirk on his face, Mr. Andrews marches to his wife's room. Their daughter told me during an interview in her home that, "He's always been like this, an authority figure."

The history of familial relationships is ever-present and can complicate negotiations with family members when crises arise.

The CNAs also have an uneasy, ambivalent relationship with Louis Feldman whose behavior thwarts the CNAs' autonomous use of their skills in caring for his wife, Edna, and disrupts the social world of the unit. A complex interactional triangle among Mr. Feldman, his wife, and Lyle Thornton, a day care member of the Pavilion, causes the husband to remain angry. One day as I observe on the Pavilion, Edna and Lyle are sitting next to one another on the couch, holding hands. CNA Chevelle expects there to be trouble if Edna's husband makes one of his unexpected visits during the day. She explains,

> Mr. Feldman, I don't think he understands what the disease is. He don't understand that she's sick. When he comes in she be like huggin' up under Lyle Thornton. They just be holding hands. One day Louis came in here and got angry and said, "Stay away from my wife." But Lyle didn't know. I don't know why he is the victim.

At the same time that Chevelle notes Mr. Feldman's intrusions on the Pavilion, she recognizes and participates in another aspect of his personality and interaction on the unit. She speaks about engaging him:

> ANNE: What do you talk to Mr. Feldman about?
>
> CHEVELLE: We just talk about making her face up real pretty and he asks me how I'm doin'. He tries to have a conversation. I kinda like that. Not in the beginning, but now.
>
> ANNE: What do you do for Edna that he likes?
>
> CHEVELLE: I just make her face up. I did it one day and she looked real pretty and he saw it and said, "Will you do that for me one day?" So I said, "I'll do it tomorrow." She was lookin' real cute. I shaved them whiskers off (gesturing by stroking her chin). She liked it.

Chevelle notes that Mr. Feldman "asks me how I'm doin'," indicating attempts on his part to recognize and engage her as person and care worker. As well, her comments imply that he has ("not at first") learned to try ("tries to make conversation") thereby bringing to light a more favorable side of Mr. Feldman. The interaction conveys respect for certain skills of the staff. LPN Marita adds her interpretation of Louis Feldman's behavior:

> He is in denial or whatever. We say that your wife—she has a right if she wants Mr. Thornton to be there. You know we will see to it that nothing happens that shouldn't happen but other than that we can't … because one day they did try to keep them separated and it agitated her so much. It's not worth—we're here for her not for him. I mean we are there to support him but our responsibility is to her.

Marita's interrupted sentence, "It's not worth … we're here for her not for him," captures the twin purposes of the CNA's care work, maintaining control and upholding their ethic of care, in this case, protecting the rights of the resident even when it goes against the wishes of the family member. Given Marita's incompletion of her first thought and immediate movement to an entirely different thought, it is reasonable to assume what she meant is "it's not worth" the disruption to staff and residents when they try to separate Edna and Lyle. This narrative connects skills and knowledge with the meaning of responsibility, a big part of the ethic. Diane's distinction between "support" and responsibility brings to the fore a tension that pervades most relationships between staff and families: Who is responsible for the resident and how is that responsibility defined? From Marita Martin and the staff's perspective, they are responsible for the resident. As CNA Chevelle states, "we are supposed to help them (residents) meet their little freedoms," which she likes. Those freedoms, however, may not be consonant with the ideas of family members.

The staff evoke moral boundaries on the Pavilion when they talk about the "rights" of residents. They assert their autonomy to decide the meaning of the situation and define behavior in the context of the specific interaction between Edna Feldman and Lyle Thornton. The philosophy tends to be laissez-faire regarding the emotional connections between residents, for example, the relationship between Boris Randolph and Carrie Mae Gordon. The CNAs respect their right to be in the room together during the day with the door ajar or closed. They tell me that Carrie Mae's family "does not have a problem with their having an intimate relationship" if they both consent. The situation with Boris and Carrie Mae is not complicated by a third party and a living spouse who comes to the Pavilion at least once a day.

Several facets of intrusions on the ethic of care and control of resident behavior are represented when conflict ensues. The CNAs are "on guard" around Louis Feldman as Carma Lee relates,

> He likes to find fault. He's never complimented us. He's always complaining, never happy. You just can't believe him. He upsets the whole unit because he is so abrupt with his wife, and when he leaves she's upset so we try and

> calm her down. When one is upset or agitated it sets off a chain reaction and before you know it you've got a whole group of people that are agitated.

According to CNA Arnella, Louis Feldman's behavior is of utmost concern to the staff whenever he visits because of their need to keep control and protect Edna's rights. She offers additional insight into how Louis comes in and berates his wife when she is sitting with Lyle Thornton.

> He yells, "Now, I don't want you to ever do that again, you hear me? You want me to come and see you? Don't you ever do that again." Like she can remember. He is in denial. He does cry, however, and says he knows that he doesn't understand. When he talks to his wife that way it gets her upset which upsets the others.

Two tendencies are evident in Arnella's account. First, she reiterates Mr. Feldman's negative effects on the unit, which hit at the heart of the CNAs' concern over control and loss of control on the Pavilion. The CNAs' ability to handle a shifting, fluid environment becomes important. They must be constantly vigilant to a heightened degree of agitation and unpredictability in residents' reactions over and above their regular watch. Second, at the same time, Arnella attributes a positive valence to Louis Feldman when she notes that "he cries, however, and knows that he doesn't understand." Arnella articulates a redeeming side of this family member in his emotional struggle with understanding the behavior of his wife. Mr. Feldman uses an argument of shaming and threats of abandonment to bring his wife around. We can turn to Goffman once again for illumination as to probable reasons for Louis Feldman's approach to his wife. Goffman[5] states:

> The constant effort for the family to argue the patient out of his foolish notions, to make him take a reasonable view—an argumentation so despaired of by some therapists—can similarly be understood as the family's need and the family's efforts to bring the patient back into appropriate relationship to them. They cannot let him have his wrong beliefs because they cannot let him go. The selves that had been the reciprocals of his are undermined. And that which should not have been able to change—the character of a loved one—appears to be changing fundamentally and for the worse right before their eyes. And life is said to become like a bad dream—for there is no place in possible realities for what is occurring.

We can understand, on another level, the provocation for Mr. Feldman's continuous berating of Edna Feldman as an attempt to shake his wife into her "rightful place" in the family and in her personal relation and duty to him as his wife. These outbursts, however, agitate other residents, create additional work for the CNAs, and are an invasion into what they regard as their rightful place to protect the "emotional well-being of the resident." The CNAs' ambivalence toward certain family members because of their disruptive activities and lack of respect for residents, including their own loved one, can be partly understood within the framework of insiders/outsiders. Mr. Feldman becomes an outsider at those moments of out-of-control behavior. Naming someone as an outsider and/or labeling a family member as a "complainer," as in the case of Mr. Feldman, allows the CNAs to anticipate behavior, thus strengthening the CNAs' locus of control over the emergence of disruption. On the other hand, the boundary between staff and family can also be lessened and mutual respect may emerge within a certain context through interaction (such as the example of Chevelle and Feldman) and the pair move a bit closer.

In another case of threats to autonomy and a contest of power, Justine points out an example of what she has been telling me about another spouse who comes on the Pavilion, Victor Turner, who "tries to run things." One day, she hurries over to me to point out Turner who is carping at Marita Martin about his wife's appearance:

> There is Mr. Turner in action. He's saying that she has no socks. As fast as we put her things up, she goes in there. We can't keep everything locked up. He comes in at different times of the day. Can't prepare for him. She was dressed real nice. Her hair combed and everything. She's changed her clothes. She's gotten in somebody else's room and got their clothes. That's not even what she had on. She was wearing one of the new blouses he bought her and everything. But he's quite upset. See, he's very angry.

It is important for Justine to verify what she has been telling me about the outbursts of Mr. Turner. Such expressions of frustration and anger are not atypical of several other families as they try to adjust to new behavior patterns in their spouse or parent. This incident gives Justine the opportunity to testify to someone, me, that the CNAs' care has been accomplished even though the family member was questioning their attention to his wife. She has a desire for me to know the truth as though to say, "this is what we are up against," an example of the usurpation of the CNAs' right to define the meaning of actions and implement their ethic of care.

An ambivalent attitude toward certain family members can heighten uncertainty. Responses to such uncertainty include developing tactics to manage their own feelings as well as manage the family members' feelings. One tactic that staff use to enhance families' understanding and foster "accepting relationships"[6] is to normalize resident behavior. Marita explains:

> We try and tell families that people's behavior doesn't bother us, that we understand and can handle it. They get upset with their family members because they act a certain way. We tell them it doesn't matter. We've seen most of those behaviors before and that is not the problem. They just get so

> upset about things. I don't know what goes on in their life but when we call them about something, it's, "I can't handle anything anymore."

With the intention of diminishing negative valence on a family member's behavior, staff use normalization as a tactic to assuage the separation between self and the loved one who has irrevocably changed.[7] When their tactics fail, Marita and her staff "set up a time for them to talk with occupational or physical therapy and sometimes that works better."

As well, normalizing a resident's behavior and respecting the rights of residents comes to light when Justine relates her response to a daughter's concerns about her mother's "mouth."

> The daughter says that the only reason they put her mother on this Pavilion was because, "We didn't like her upstairs in the nursing home because my mother can be, you could say, quite abusive with her mouth." I said, "Well she can be, but we know how to handle that. We can deal with that. You know she can say anything she wants to—she's 100 years old. I don't care what she says to me."

Staffs' ambivalence, which can turn into understanding and a positive relationship, occurs with resident Grace Nicholson's family. A pattern of intrusions by Grace's family concerns lying to Grace when the family has to end their visit and leave. LPN Carma Lee describes the emotional situation for all concerned:

> Grace's family went through a time when they would leave and would lie to her. She would say, "I'm not crazy but they think I am because they stuck me in a home." It made the staff feel so bad. We told the family that, "it not only affects her (Grace) it affects us." So we told them just to tell her you have to go because she's adjusted quite well. She knows when they come they have to leave. But just don't lie to her. Don't have us to take her away and just sneak off. That upsets her and she has a really bad day. The last time it was just too hard for us all, too hard. Every one of us would do something different with her to try to cheer her up and nothing worked. So we told Marita to call the family and tell them this is not good for her—we were all crying. So they came the other day and told her they were coming and when they had to leave. She was just fine and hugged her husband. I was so happy. She's *not* crazy.

The staff think a great deal of Grace Nicholson. She is one of their favorites and they have come to respect her family. One day I asked CNA Chevelle what came to her mind when I mentioned a series of residents. When we came to Grace, Chevelle paused for a moment. "She be her name."

Similar to what Carma Lee emphasizes, LPN Marita Martin also emphasizes the importance of not lying in the following:

> I think that's the biggest success with the unit—never lie. Don't lie about something. No matter, don't. Boy, that's the worst thing you can do. Because someone's going to come along and lie for you. I don't do lies. If you're going to do something and you're going to execute it, do it correctly. You can make a mistake, come back and tell me. We can mend it someway. It's not that you meant to do it. It wasn't intentional. Don't (lie) because you're going to pay the piper sooner or later.

In her longitudinal study of a caregiver's support group for Alzheimer families, Nancy Blum[8] investigates how family members learn and use deceptive practices to convince family members to accept and voluntarily go along with control efforts. Blum[9] argues that in the case of the Alzheimer family, deceptive practices have become a way of life. She explains,

> It is tied to the details of daily living, namely, accomplishing tasks and maintaining some semblance of order in the household. Whereas the utilization of deception in other contexts revolves around the control of information, in the Alzheimer's case, it serves the end of informal social control, that is, managing a family member's behavior.

Families in Blum's[10] study use deception on a regular basis to avoid what she calls "potential troublesome action" from a family member. Similarly, the CNAs use their knowledge to circumvent and outwit potential family and resident behavior that creates a level of agitation affecting the Pavilion as a whole. There is, however, a significant difference between the *amount* of deceptive practice in a collective setting such as the Alzheimer's Pavilion and in the primary group setting. With jobs and multiple responsibilities, the families in Blum's study have a "second shift"[11] of caring for their family member with Alzheimer's disease. Thus, the families' ubiquitous use of what Blum refers to as "little white lies" becomes necessary for management of the aberrant behavior of their loved one in the home setting.

In contrast, the Starrmount Alzheimer's staff's official full-time job *is* care work. While CNAs may use "little white lies" from time to time, other strategies to control resident behavior while promoting emotional well-being predominate on the Pavilion. Deception is not a way of life on the Pavilion for several reasons. The Alzheimer's staff are paid (though not nearly enough) to provide care and they have initiated what we have come to understand as a "different" care. Some of their time can be directed toward discovery work such as observing the behavior of Miss Ava making beds, finding out why she gets into fights with another resident, and developing strategies to prevent such outbursts. The staff, as semi-professional care workers, do not have the kind, or length, of relational history with the residents that family members do, with its latent and manifest intentions. CNAs work at creating a new relationship with the residents, by recognizing the emergence of "the new self." As well, in the home, there is not the group socializing that can happen in a collective setting. Because of their use of relative autonomy, the latitude with which staff can allow resident "trouble" expands; disruptions on the Pavilion are expected as part of the daily existence and are folded into the whole.

"That's All We're Supposed To Know"

Many families hold stereotypical views of CNAs; they devaluate CNAs' knowledge and range of skills, treating them as "social invisibles," on the unit. CNA Justine's comments are representative of all CNAs' sentiments regarding family members' view of staff: "The families think that all we do is keep them clean and fed and looking nice. That's all we're supposed to know. I think it should change. I really do." With the exception of two or three families I interviewed who do recognize the CNAs' knowledge, Justine's contention is right on the mark for the rest of the families. She gives an example:

> I try to explain to them what happens. I say, "I'll tell you what. Let me go get Marita." Sometimes they feel like maybe we just don't know what we are talking about, the aides. Or we're just making up an excuse or something. I'll try to explain the best that I can, but I always say, "Let me get the nurse."

While affirming the concern and kindness of the staff, a number of family members hold stereotypical views of CNAs as very limited in skills and intelligence. The levels of reflection and subtlety are brought forth in the Starrmount CNAs' thinking, and their array of skills demonstrated in this study challenge such thinking. One of the manifestations of this attitude is family members rebuffing, ignoring or challenging the staff (and going to LPN, Marita Martin) which Arnella describes: "Sometimes family members will walk right up to you and *by* you and will not speak to you." Thus, families' and visitors' assumptions of lack of knowledge can extend to lack of *acknowledgment*. While I did not hear family members make racists remarks to or about the CNAs, RN Elaine Pressley tells me that it was not uncommon for families to state unequivocally, "I don't want that 'Black one' touching my family member."

The feeling of elitism coming from some family members as to the paucity of a CNA's knowledge can extend upward to those higher in the bureaucratic hierarchy, as RN Elaine Pressley relates:

> Harriet French is a very busy person. Always walking. Into things, picking up things. We have difficulty with her family. I really don't know how realistic

> they are about the disease process. It's like, "Mother doesn't do those things. Mother wouldn't do this." Oh yes, she would. They tell you they understand. Like she takes her shoes and socks off. We find them all kinds of places. They're upset because they're missing. We want her to wear her glasses and they tried new glasses on her today and she won't wear them. It's like they say they know about the disease but they don't really. I don't know if they accept the reality of it. Also, I have the feeling and Marita does too, it's like when they're talking to you, they're looking down their noses at you. Helen falls a lot. My feeling is that they don't always believe what you tell them. Maybe you're doing something to make her fall.

Elaine's experience supports the CNA's view of how some families regard them. Underscoring the importance of nuances in social interaction, Elaine explains, "It's not so much what they (family members) say, it's *how* they say it." Distrust on both sides coupled with what the staff perceive as expressions of class differentiation exacerbate the already existing tension in relationships with certain families. Staff may ignore these families when they come to the Pavilion given their relational history. Such a strategy helps to protect their autonomy to choose engagement or not, as well as protect them from the strain of confrontations.

Concerning Elaine Pressley's claim that the family is "in denial" about their mother's condition, we can draw again on Goffman[12] who provides additional insight into possible reasons for the stance:

> The claims and actions of the ill person are not necessarily bizarre in themselves, merely bizarre when coming from the particular patient addressing himself to this particular family. And bizarreness is not the issue. Even when the patient hallucinates or develops exotic beliefs, the concern of the family is not simply that a member has crazy notions but that he is not keeping his place in relationships. Someone to whom we are closely related is someone who ought not to have beliefs or actions which estrange him from us.

According to RN Pressley, the family is resolute in their position that Helen would never take her shoes and socks off and hide them everywhere; not wear the newly purchased glasses by her family, what could be termed "bizarre" behavior from Goffman's perspective. These images of Helen are not ones that are consistent with the view of their mother's place within the family. To accept such behavior as coming from her would severely test, if not crush the family's perspective.

Prefacing her comments with, "I know this is a silly thing but …," RN Elaine Pressley expresses her exasperation with families who call about feeding their family member:

> They'll come in over the weekend and they will ask, "do you feed her?" My first inclination is to say, "No. No we don't." It just ticks you off. We

> have families that come in every night to feed their family and if they're not coming they'll call and say, "I can't be there tonight. Will you have somebody feed her?" You want to say, "No, if you don't come, they don't eat." I know that's a silly thing but it just ticks me off.

While RN Elaine Pressley claims these inquiries are a "silly thing," her tone is one of indignation when the issue of responsibility for the resident's well-being, to say nothing of their basic needs, comes into question. It's almost as if she wants to shout, "What the hell do you think we are doing here?"

The CNAs have an easy and close relationship with two African American families. Justine expresses her agency by explaining and giving an example of one standard of interpersonal behavior which they see as meeting the staff's need for respect and recognition. She offers an interpersonal model of communication that promotes emotional well-being for both staff and residents:

> Take Gloria Reynolds (Miss Ava's daughter). She's here three or four times a week. She comes to the CNAs and makes us feel important and like we know what's going on. She talks to us and asks questions. And after we try to explain what's happening with Miss Ava, Gloria then goes to see Marita and says the "girls told me such and such."

Justine gives words to a model of behavior that embodies one part of the staff's behavioral expectations for everyone on the Pavilion. Habermas[13] provides insight into the consequences of such recognition through his concept of "two different modes of employing language" (author's emphases):

> In one mode of language use, *one says what is or is not the case.* In the other, *one says something to someone else in a way that allows him to understand what is being said.* Only the second mode of language use is internally or conceptually tied up with the conditions of communication. Saying how things stand does not necessarily depend on any kind of real or imagined communication; one does not need to *make* a statement, that is, perform a speech act. When we are dealing with a purely cognitive, non-communicative use of language, only *one* fundamental relation is involved: Let us call it the relationship between sentences and something in the world *about* which the sentences state something. In contrast, when language is used for coming to terms or reaching an understanding with someone else (even if it is ultimately only to agree or disagree), three relations are involved: by giving an expression *of* his belief, the speaker communicates *with* another member of the same speech community *about* something in the world.

Justine's model of interaction between Gloria Reynolds and the CNAs indicates the three relations of which Habermas speaks: (1) Gloria assumes (believes) that the CNAs are deserving of respect and that they are knowledgeable (an expression *of* her belief); (2) She talks with them and asks how they are (communicating *with* the CNAs as members of the same speech community); (3) Gloria asks questions of the CNAs to understand how her mother is doing. Assuming that the CNAs' interpretations are credible, she takes their understandings to Marita Martin as a foundation to obtain more information if necessary (communicating *about* something in the world). In fact, there are *two* communication levels going on simultaneously here: language used as communication *about* the CNAs ("She (Gloria) makes us feel important, like we know what's going on") as well as language used as communication *about* Gloria's mother ("what's happening with Miss Ava"). Other CNAs echo the "good" communication between themselves and Miss Ava's daughter, Gloria, as a standard of interpersonal behavior and interaction. In this regard, Habermas's second form of communication helps but is not fully adequate to understand the details when applied in this case.

Both Gloria Reynolds and Rachel Price, Boots' daughter, relate well to the CNAs. In an interview, Rachel Price, an executive with a fast-paced life and much responsibility, speaks of going to the Alzheimer's Pavilion "to relax and unwind" because she enjoys being there with all the residents. She speaks about the "intimacy" she feels with the CNAs and Marita Martin and what they know about her family's life:

> I helped (on the Pavilion) by initially sitting with the residents. So, they (staff) came to know when Randy (son) calls from Tokyo or when Billy (son) calls from L.A. They've gotten to know the family so well that when my sister showed up last Christmas from St. Louis they called and said, "Ah, do you have a sister? (big laugh) Wel-l-l-l-l, she-e-e-e's here." You know when I really think about it we're all pretty intimate. This has absolutely become extended family. Early on they would take Boots to church. Justine did that and kinda gloated about it like, "I've got Verna for Christmas Eve." I can't imagine any family member not feeling like I feel.

At the same time, from another perspective, Carma Lee is cautious about coming to understandings with families:

> I don't know, for some reason I feel like some of these family members think that we can work miracles—which we can't. It does make your work that much harder when you have family members thinking, "Oh, my loved one is going to get better because they're in here"—because they're not.

Carma expresses a possible contradiction in her thinking. In other interviews and informal discussions with her, she spoke of her delight "when the resident progressed even just an inch."

In large part, Marita and her staff articulate, monitor and maintain the Pavilion's "ethic of care." As I have shown above, the narrative of daily life on the Pavilion reveals that this normative structure includes: enhancing the emotional well-being of residents; practicing respect for all residents as a behavioral principle; protecting the rights of individual residents and "helping them meet their little freedoms" even when it may go against family wishes; preserving dimensions of resident self; and, trying to keep the resident's mind "workin'."

Notes

1 Specific aspects of the staff ethic of care include enhancing the wellbeing of residents; practicing respect for all residents as a behavioral principle; protecting the rights of individual residents, and "helping them meet their little freedoms" even when it may go against family wishes; preserving dimensions of the resident self; and, trying to keep the resident's "mind workin'." For insightful works on the ethics of care see: Annemarie Mol, *The Logic of Care: Health and the Problem of Patient Choice* (London: Routledge, 2006); Marian Barnes, *Care in Everyday Life: An Ethics of Care in Practice* (Bristol: The Policy Press, 2012); and, Marian Barnes and Tula Brannelly (eds) *Ethics of Care: Critical Advances in International Perspective* (Bristol: The Policy Press, 2015).

2 Robert Bogdan and Steven Carter, "The Social Construction of Humanness: Relationships with Severely Disabled People," *Interpreting Disability: A Qualitative Reader* 7(1992): 275–294.

3 Erving Goffman, "The Insanity of Place," *Psychiatry: Journal for the Study of Interpersonal Processes* XXXII (1969): 362.

4 Ibid., 362.

5 Ibid., 366.

6 Robert Bogdan and Steven Taylor, "Toward a Sociology of Acceptance: The Other Side of the Study of Deviance," *Social Policy* 18 (1987): 3.

7 For more on relations between husbands and spouses when the female has Alzheimer's disease see: Jeanne Hayes, Craig Boylstein and Mary K. Zimmerman, "Living and Loving with Dementia: Negotiating Spousal and Caregiver Identity Through Narrative," *Journal of Aging Studies* 23 (2009): 48–59, and, Jeanne Hayes, Mary K. Zimmerman and Craig Boylstein, "Responding to Symptoms of Alzheimer's Disease: Husbands, Wives, and the Gendered Dynamics of Recognition and Disclosure," *Qualitative Health Research* 20 (2010): 1101–1115.

8 Nancy Blum, "Deceptive Practices in Managing a Family Member with Alzheimer's Disease," *Symbolic Interaction* 17 (1994): 21–36.

9 Ibid., 22.

10 Ibid., 27.

11 Arlie Hochschild, *The Second Shift: Working Parents and the Revolution at Home* (New York: Viking Penguin, 1989). Also, Robert Emerson and Sheldon Messinger, "The Micro-Politics of Trouble," *Social Problems* 25 (1977): 122.

12 Erving Goffman, "The Insanity of Place," *Psychiatry: Journal for the Study of Interpersonal Processes*, XXXII (1969): 362.

13 Jürgen Habermas, *Moral Consciousness and Communicative Action* (Cambridge, MA: The MIT Press, 1991): 24.

7

"WE'RE NOT A ZOO"

After lunch, the lights dim for a peaceful interlude called "quiet time" on the Alzheimer's Pavilion. The hustle and bustle of the noon hour is turning into a languid afternoon when the large entry doors open and a group of six people, some clad in white coats, stride into the Pavilion. Today's group of five from a local university medical school stop, as though locked in space, at the boundary of the sitting area to survey the residents from a distance. Part of a teaching hospital, groups of interns and medical personnel come to the Pavilion on a regular basis. From the staff's perspective, however, they never step into the world of even a minimal understanding of those they observe. RN Elaine Pressley's candor captures staff members' sentiments about such visits when she comments,

> The medical students come and some could care less if they are here. It's not their bag—they're going to be a surgeon or OBGYN and the thing that makes me mad is they make no bones about this. You just want to say, "Then don't be here."[1]

Justine wastes no time in advancing toward them. "May I help you?" she asks. The CEO of Starrmount Geriatric thanks her but says the guests have heard about the Pavilion and he is taking them around to see a resident's room. The staff do not offer to talk with the guests and the guests do not ask any questions of the staff. Instead, they turn to the CEO to ask about the Pavilion. Justine moves backward to attend to a resident but keeps her eyes nailed on the group. Interaction between Marita and the group is polite but minimal, enough to do her duty. Heads are up behind the nurses' alcove and Marita Martin continues to work on her "interminable" paperwork. As I watch Marita and know that she is all ears, I think of her disgust at the aloofness of such groups who come to "gaze":[2]

MARITA: I get upset because we're not a zoo. You don't come in my unit and stare at my people because they're not animals. They're not on display.

ANNE: When and how would this happen?

MARITA: They come in and they would just stand and stare.

ANNE: "They" meaning?

MARITA: The group. Let's say the United Way or medical students come in. They would come in at breakfast time or maybe lunch and just stare. Like we were different. I don't like that.

ANNE: Is that typical behavior of someone who comes in?

MARITA: I think so. I know their interests may be to benefit the unit. But it just gives you a sense of, "you came in to look at us like we were not ok." Let me not say this word. See, I'm thinking in my own Alzheimer's thoughts.

ANNE: OK. Explain that.

MARITA: That's like, when I'm in there, I think with and for the residents, so I'm almost whatever it is, I'm in that world for eight hours, sometimes sixteen. Whatever it is. It's ok for you to mumble, to come and garble at me. It's ok because I'm going to try and understand what it is that you're trying to tell me. I want to say that for me that's normal. For me it's normal because I work with them every day. But to them ("outsiders" as staff refer to these visiting groups) it's not normal, it's abnormal. So they want to see what the "hubbub" is about.

Noteworthy in LPN Marita's remarks is the use of the inclusive "we." Injury to the residents is injury to Marita and the CNAs. Her language about outsiders and medical students, "They come in and just stand and stare … and look at us like we were not ok," express the staff's sentiments precisely. Being "not ok" means that activities and practices of the Pavilion are not standardized and regulated by bureaucratic rules. The staff's aversion to spectators' "ways of seeing," absent of understanding, can become contentious.

Ways of Seeing: The Medical Model and the State

I am sitting in the blue chairs taking notes and listening to residents Roy, Boris, and Carrie Mae. They are laughing and focusing on Mr. Randolph's shoes as CNA Chevelle listens. Without warning, a female physician almost lights on Carrie Mae's shoulder, peers over her and says:

DOC: Hello, I'm Dr. Trumble Can you tell me how old you are? (decontextualizing)

CARRIE MAE: (looks around as if to say who is this?) Wha-at? (mumbling, when before she had been clear)

DOC: What is your name?

CARRIE MAE: (with a quizzical smile, looks up and stares at the doctor)

DOC: (undeterred and moving right along) Who is the president of the United States? By now, Carrie Mae is bewildered at this line of questioning. The doctor says a cheery "Thank you," pivots, and leaves the Pavilion with the official chart in hand.

ANNE: (turning to look at Carrie Mae) You look like you're deep in thought.

CARRIE MAE: (as if to show the best of her capacities in contrast to what had occurred and with a different smile and sarcastic tone). I am, but what good will it do ...? What can I do with it ...?

With that, Carrie Mae raises her hands in front of her, punctuated with an impish smile as if to confirm the reality of what had transpired. Somehow she sensed the Catch 22 and the irony of it all—encounter, not engagement. CNA Chevelle, annoyed, whispers, "We don't like the way they don't respect the residents by asking them those questions out of the blue. She could see they were having a conversation." According to Chevelle, this disrespect happens on a regular basis.

The voice of medicine and the scientific attitude meet the voice of the life world and the natural attitude of everyday life in this exchange. The physician imposes upon Carrie Mae a frame within which she must respond. Carrie Mae's reaction is one of puzzlement. The physician came to Carrie Mae not as person, but as a patient with a label—Alzheimer's patient, passive without agency. The inability to put oneself in the role or attitude of the other leads to a misunderstanding of the behavior of the resident. Through the lens of the medical model, Carrie Mae's reactions are seen as signs and symptoms of the disease, rather than her attempts to make sense out of the situation. As a result, the self and personal identity of Carrie Mae are not confirmed.

In refraining from answering Dr. Trumble, Carrie Mae fulfills the expectation of the medical model corroborating her disorientation. The physician considers herself competent and humane; however, she is unable to move into the resident's world. The view of residents as property, with access assumed, characterizes the physicians' approach more times than not. The hegemony of physicians, and the subjugation of the CNAs' body of knowledge, pose threats to the autonomous functioning of the Pavilion on a regular basis.

Staff's strategy for maintaining a degree of autonomy in the midst of intrusion by physicians is a polite disengagement. While they cannot control entry and exit to the Pavilion, they can control *access* to their world. Starrmount administrators have full rights to come on the Pavilion and do whatever they choose to showcase it as a model. The "strategic" space that the CNAs have created can become *contested* space when these intrusions occur. Marita Martin frames the encounter between the staff and visitors as oppositional when she apprises me that "We are very territorial." She goes on to say, "I don't like gawkers and I politely go through the motions just to get them off of the unit." During one of our interviews, Marita Martin relates a phone conversation which, while not typical of every physician, is not unusual: "The Physician asked, 'What do you do here?'" "I answered, 'I'm the Licensed Practical Charge Nurse.'" "Then the doc said, 'I want to talk to a *real* nurse.'"

> ANNE: Will they use those words?
>
> MARITA: Oh, yeah. A real nurse. We know what they mean, an RN. I said, "Well, I'm sorry. They're at lunch right now. You're going to have to talk to me." You have to get to them and then that's not good. It's not good rapport.
>
> ANNE: What happens then?
>
> MARITA: He had to give it to me, whatever it is. I didn't go to school for nothing. But they do talk to you like you're just an idiot and you don't know what you are talking about. Now some of them, they'll go as far as whatever you need.

The physician acts out the meaning of professional dominance as he attempts to put Marita in her place. Marita's response to this power assertion is to stand pat and force an interaction. She refuses to acquiesce by leaving a message for a "real" nurse. CNA Arnella recognizes the issue of occupational licensing and makes her own case as to who knows more about the residents:

> Well, I don't have that LPN title, RN title behind my name, so I can't know. I don't know as much as they know. Granted I don't, but when it comes to these residents, we know more than they do because we're working with them one on one every day.

Theirs is a "privileged" knowledge in the sense that Habermas argues: "Knowledge becomes privileged because it is based on lived experience to which individuals have privileged access."[3]

It is not uncommon for physicians to construct status differences through such interaction and devalue the lower ranks of health care workers. Physicians usually rush into the Pavilion and head for the nurse's alcove. They read patient's charts, check for "reality-orientation" as in the case of Carrie Mae Gordon, and attend to medical problems that are out of the purview of staff but are not serious enough for hospital treatment. The visit is perfunctory and part of a routinized agenda with minimal interaction with the staff unless there has been an emergency.

The power of the institution of medicine, in conjunction with the state's licensing power emanates from the capacity to define identity.[4] Identity in this sense refers to what Arnella says is "having that LPN, RN title behind my name" not CNA. Thus, the CNAs' occupational identity precludes their inscribing in the chart because their knowledge is deemed ineligible. The authority to define what knowledge *can be inscribed* in the chart rests with the medical institution and the state. It is important to keep in mind that CNAs do not own the right to *officially* control knowledge in the same way as those above them in the hierarchy. On the one hand, the staff's claims to privileged knowledge are valid for the reasons stated. On the other hand, knowledge is defined and legitimated by RNs and the physicians who have power over others. CNAs are labeled as "not knowing" by virtue of what they are *not*, RNs or LPNs.

The CNAs' knowledge, in relation to "official" knowledge, could be considered a "naïve or disqualified knowledge, beneath the required level of cognition or scientificity."[5] Here is what is *crucial*, however: Whether claims by the staff of a different, exclusive knowledge are justified (if that were possible to determine), is not the issue. Their *identity* derived from a privileged concept is. Their frustration in not having it recognized is evident. We need to go beyond Foucault's argument about the social fact or condition of CNAs' knowledge as disqualified. The staff *act* on this identity, maintain the script and assert it in their work. The identity of being special and having different knowledge of the residents is a source of pride and motivation as well as frustration, because of lack of recognition. The staff think of themselves as both "specialist" in their knowledge of the residents, and "special" in their caregiving and relating to the residents. While this identity is accomplished in large part through relative autonomy, it is also threatened by the same.

Charting

Frustration with the chart comes to light when CNA Justine reveals important material that is absent both from resident Alice Duncan's chart and the discussion at the Plan of Care Meeting[6] with the family. The CNA's concern is to increase the emotional well-being of Alice as Justine relates:

> I just hate writin' some stuff on some paper enough to live with the state or whoever. We want to see Alice (a resident) doing something. We want to get her motivated here and get her to start doing some things and talking with us. If you don't say anything to her she won't say anything to you. We want to be able to be in this plan of care conference and program and have our say in this planning of care thing. Ms. Pressley comes and asks me: "Justine." and I say, "Uh huh." "Does Alice feed herself? Does she go to the bathroom? How does she know she gets her bath?" Well you need to know that. You shouldn't have to come to me. So I feel if you're going to come to me and ask all those questions and I give you all those answers—why shouldn't I be in the meeting? I might as well be.

Justine makes a distinction between "stuff" (categories) constructed by medical and bureaucratic entities to meet official guidelines, and what the CNAs can tell them about Alice's care. The CNAs question why their skills and knowledge are not part of the decision-making process and the discussion about resident Alice

Duncan. Marita Martin told me in confidence that the reason they (the administrative staff) don't want Justine in the Plan of Care meetings was because she "tells it like it is." Justine tells me that she did attend one Plan of Care Meeting and "nothing was being done" which coincides with Marita's reason for not attending. Whether or not the evaluation of such meetings is valid or not, the CNAs' *perception* is important in coloring their view of administration. Thus, authority over what is chosen as knowledge about a resident can affect the care work and day-to-day operation of the Pavilion in two fundamental ways. First, it can provide a measure of power over current, as well as subsequent treatment of the residents. Second, in the case of oral knowledge, it can strengthen the idea of autonomy on the Pavilion, free of structural restraints from the outside. The reality, however, is that this knowledge remains "hidden." Power to create categories, power to define what is important in the care of residents, and power to inscribe the breadth and depth of the care work that challenges the routinization of the medical model is denied official recognition.

The CNAs' autonomy to construct meaning in their own terms and have their knowledge of residents entered into the official record is disrupted in the case of the patient chart. The chart has no categories for what CNAs consider to be their different knowledge. The cold reality is if it's not documented, it didn't happen. Therefore, the CNAs' defense against threats to their autonomy and knowledge of the residents is to build a reservoir of oral knowledge, which they pass to one another. Moreover, while inscription of their knowledge of the residents is curtailed by definitions imposed from the macro-environment, this "knowledge in practice" is the fundamental medium for social interaction in the Alzheimer's Pavilion. It is perpetuated and preserved through "speaking the knowledge" in an oral tradition.

As an official document, the chart symbolizes the ultimate in social control. Resident self is invisible and "bed and body work" is writ large. Recording of bed making, bathing schedule, bowel and bladder regimen, weights and vital signs throughout the day, constitute charting. Each function is treated as discrete which separates the gestalt of the whole person. What is missing from the chart is a distinctive part of the CNAs' ethic of care, the attendance to the "emotional well-being" of the resident as it is intertwined with physical care. Its absence leaves a truncated record of the functions of a body not the life of a human being.

The fact that the staff's different knowledge is not recorded in the charts is very important. It is an example of how the institution classifies individuals and confers a synoptic identity through the chart. The chart limits what can be inscribed about a "patient," separating what is necessary to be done (body inventory) from what is not. Selective recording means a biased (by the dominant medical model discourse) re-presentation and construction of life on the Pavilion. A totality of care is being provided but it is not inscribed nor recognized. When the CNAs talk about their perceptions of the residents, I ask them where this was recorded. Smiling, one CNA takes her index finger and taps on her head, "Up here, we have it." Arnella addresses the question of whether CNAs write comments in the resident charts:

> (shaking her head) No, we tell Marita (the charge nurse). But it is information that she needs and it may be small to you and me but not to the family. The charge nurse can't be everywhere. *We have to be her eyes and ears.* We have good communication with the charge nurse even if we ourselves don't write it in the chart. If you don't know all these little things then you can't pass them on and something might go wrong. They wouldn't know about these things that happen. The staff fill each other in.

The privileged nature of the CNAs' knowledge is given support through Arnella's noting that the CNAs are the Charge Nurse's "eyes and ears." The Certified Nursing Assistants have a certain amount of power in that it is they who choose what is relevant information about the residents; however, there is a "catch-22." That power is compromised because the chart defines and delimits the categories. The fact that the knowledge is oral requires a different set of abilities to recall and use. Oral knowledge is kept alive and reconstructed by passing it on to teammates, testing it out, and amending again. The literature on frontline workers does not typically acknowledge such levels of reflection nor recognize their empowering consequences for a group of workers who have had little or no voice historically.

Since Marita Martin and the CNAs think of the residents as a second family, they enjoy talking about the different personalities that make up the Pavilion. They have given residents nicknames based on traits they have observed. Carrie Mae Gordon is "Cookie" or "Cookie Monster" because, as Arnella tells me, "This woman loves cookies of all kinds." "Ruby Klein is 'Miss Vogue,' a woman who likes fashion and manners," according to Carma Lee. "Softball," is Marge Jacobs, one of the favorites of the staff. Marge's constant chant, "Out goes she into the deep blue sea, softball seven eleven," echoes throughout the Pavilion. Alice is "The Boss" because she needs to be in charge. Verna Jarret is "Boots" because that is the name she is known by and also because she "really has it going on, struttin' her stuff and so fun-lovin'," as Justine explains:

> Resident Verna Jarret, her nickname is "Boots." When you call her "Boots" it tickles her. And the State came in and they didn't want to hear us call the residents nothing but by their name. And it upset us because it was so formal and this is our home away from home. This is our family (said with emphasis) away from family and we don't feel comfortable and nor do they. Cause, sometimes they will tell us, "Oh, Honey you don't have to call me … just call me this or that," and it makes them feel comfortable and we were pretty upset with that. They call us "honey," "sweetie," sometimes they call me "fatso." That doesn't bother me because they call me "fats" at

> home. It doesn't bother me at all. We just gotta be comfortable and make the residents comfortable.[7]

Staff take umbrage at the dictates of the state inspection team because it threatens "our home away from home" (the Pavilion) and the right to "do family." The CNAs see this action of the state as an assault on the intimacy between staff and residents and the CNAs' social construction of resident individuality and identity through colorful nicknames. As a rationalized entity, the state wants to standardize behavior not particularize it, which is the antithesis of the staff's approach.

When Nursing Home Inspectors are on the Pavilion, Carma Lee reacts to an intrusion by feeling pressured to have the residents make a positive impression, which is taxing:

> Sometimes it can be demanding when different ones come in—we have a lot of students that come in from like the university medical center to observe so sometimes it is. You know they're like I was telling you about their room situation … they're going to tear up and they always seem like they sense when someone's there and that's when they really are at work, it seems like. Well you might say like children. They wait until someone comes or when you're on the phone that's when they tend to act up. That's how they are and you know how they are—trying to keep them calm and keep yourself calm so yes, it can be kind of demanding.

On one occasion, a resident takes matters into her own hands when an intrusion occurs. State Inspectors appear on the Pavilion when the residents are getting ready to participate in one of their activities. When resident Ruby Kline spots the inspectors she squares her shoulders, stands her ground, and yells: "How dare you do this to my store. Nobody asked me if you could do this. Get out of here." Ruby may or may not be referring to her family-owned department store of long ago, but reacting to a felt intrusion into the life world of the Pavilion. For an instant, the levity provided by Ruby's unwitting defense of autonomy helps to temper the dehumanizing effects of the inspection process for the CNAs.

Ways of Seeing: Bureaucracy and its Agents

Lunch is over and the CNAs are assisting some residents to their seats in the family room. Other residents are walking around, engaged in animated talk about the live turtle that was on the unit earlier in the morning. He enthralled the residents. As I look back at the now deserted dining table, I am fascinated by resident Annie Coleman's actions. With deliberation, she goes over to one of the small side tables where towels are stacked and selects one from the center. Unfolding it, she moves to the end of the long dining table. She grabs the cloth, and rubs the table. Extending her arms, she takes a series of swaths moving across the surface, and steps back to take a look at her handiwork. I catch an ever-so-slight smile of satisfaction playing at the corners of her mouth. Right away she plies her trade to another segment of the table, all the time absorbed in the work. "Oh no," comes from my right and I see Arnella advancing toward Annie. She puts her arm around her shoulders and says, "You don't have to do this today." Annie looks up and says, "But I'd rather." Arnella sighs and takes the cloth from her hand and coaxes Annie, who looks bewildered, back to the sitting area to sit with her friend, Ruby. Later that afternoon when Arnella has a free moment, I ask her why she had to stop Annie from wiping the table. Shaking her head, as though upset, she explains:

> After the residents eat, we take away all the trays. Annie would always wash the tables. It was good therapy for her. She wasn't bothering anybody. She was enjoying it and she looked forward to doing it. She's not hurting anybody and nobody is hurting her. But administration came one day when she was cleaning and they told us she was not to do it anymore. They never gave us a reason why. So we had to cut back on how much she did it.

Using opportunities for "keeping the residents' minds workin'" is integral to the staff's ethic. One day, Annie, a former waitress and domestic worker, picked up the towel to clean after lunch. The CNAs' recognition of the value of Annie's urge to clean is an indicator of two things. First it speaks to the staff's focus on using residents' understandings (getting into the resident's world) as the impetus for their care work strategies. That is, Annie's pleasure is the barometer of cleaning as "therapy." Second, such activity serves the practical purpose of keeping a resident focused on productive action, thus diminishing levels of agitation for the residents as a whole. As Carma Lee says, Annie is "feisty" and can stir up the group. Administration's infringement on the CNAs' autonomy is evident because the application of their skills is unnoticed, unappreciated and negated without explanation.

"I Will Kick Your Ass": Staff

Intrusions can come from any level of the institutional hierarchy. Marita Martin defends autonomy after a housekeeper reported her impressions of work activity in the Pavilion. Marita explains:

> We were reported by one of the housekeepers, but she's not "all there" anyway. She went and told somebody in the office that all we do is sit around and watch television and that's all we do down here. I was very offended about it. Of course I had to go talk to that individual. I said, "You know, you haven't the slightest idea of what's going on here." This is the type of person you have to deal with roughly and I said, "I will kick your ass." I'm glad it wasn't Mr. Greenberg (to whom the housekeeper spoke).

I ask her what she thinks CEO Greenberg's reaction would be. "He wouldn't have believed it. He knows how we are. He knows how much stamina we have and how much we care about the unit. This is his baby. He gave birth to it."

Justine questions the staffing coordinator's information about technical work records and defends autonomy in the chain of command. Being candid, as one comes to expect from Justine Jackson, she says:

> She's (staffing coordinator) a liar and she comes and tells us things and we have to go over her head to Allison Brown (Nursing Supervisor) to check it out. She and I are always clashing because I told her she can't tell me anything and expect me to sit back and take it. I'm gonna ask especially when you're talking about my money, my vacation days. She gets mad when I go over her head to Allison. I told her she was playing games with people. I don't bite my tongue with her, Greenberg, any of 'em.

Justine told me that she had "always been outspoken" but working in the Alzheimer's unit for six years she has become "even more outspoken." Marita Martin tells me that she worries about what she thinks are the manifestations of stress in Justine who has "killer migraines" which come from a "bad situation in her family." Contrary to some, Marita Martin argues that struggles outside the Pavilion make the CNAs stronger and more able to understand the suffering of the residents. When I asked Arnella to describe a bad day she did not have to think twice:

> When other people come on the Pavilion and aggravate our residents. As a matter of fact they put a memo out that said that there was too much traffic in and out of the Alzheimer's Pavilion. People would walk through our door and unit to go to the third unit and they didn't want them doing it because it's disruptive. I guess some people disregarded it because it still happens. You know we have a TV in the living room. They may come and stand right in front of the TV and Henrietta will tell them, "Move, I'm trying to watch TV." She has every right to watch TV and they shouldn't come and stand in front of it because they are interested in what's going on at that time (said with anger). Marita has told some people, "don't come through here."

After several complaints from the staff, administration issued a memo on unnecessary traffic coming through the Alzheimer's Pavilion. According to the CNAs, the memo has not deterred some from using the unit as a shortcut to the third unit. As though wanting to emphasize the validity and importance of the staff's complaints, Arnella's choice of words convey that, "as a matter of fact," administration (as authority with legitimate power) does not sanction such behavior.

Justine provides another insight into intrusions of outside staff into the life world of the Pavilion. When I arrived one Tuesday morning around 9:00 I noticed

Justine and an unidentified worker in a white coat in conversation. Later, I came to know that Justine was defending a resident's right to sleep, as well as the CNAs' *right* to let her sleep, to a house supervisor from another floor, an "outsider."

STAFF OUTSIDER: Well, I don't see Marge up and Roy up this morning?

JUSTINE: They're not up because they don't want to be up. She wants to sleep. She will be up before lunch. Don't worry about it.

STAFF OUTSIDER: (persistent in her tone) Well, is that good for them?

JUSTINE: (whirling around to face the outsider) Listen, I tell you what you do. You go in there and discuss getting up with her. You go in there and discuss giving him a bath. You do it because we know. Don't be coming and telling anything about our people over here because we know how they act. When that first approach is made then you've got to wait. You've got to wait and then you go back and approach them again differently. We're not going to drag them. They have rights. We are not going to violate any of their rights. So if she doesn't want to get up or if she's not going to eat her breakfast right now then we're not going to make her do that because she has the right to refuse. We'll go back later. When you want to know something, you ask us *first* what's going on.

The conversation is halted when the outsider is paged to her floor. Turning to me, Justine says, "I know it's gonna be a bad day when somebody comes over here and tells us a thing about our people early in the morning, someone from outside the unit, an outsider."

Justine's response to an outsider's intrusion on the CNA's autonomy can be interpreted on several levels as she constructs her case for "different" care by re-framing the issue on her own terms. First, she conveys the level of difficulty inherent in convincing some residents to get out of bed or take a bath by challenging the house supervisor to do it herself. Implicit in her statement is the notion that there might be good reasons why they sleep "late." Second, she follows the challenge interactionally with a description of a well-considered strategy the CNAs use. Third, Justine brings to bear the rights of residents, one of which is to sleep "late." "We are not going to violate any of their rights," she asserts. Thus, she weds two concerns of the CNAs in their work, getting the residents to do what they need for them to do and providing person-centered, humane care. When I posed the same question to other CNAs they gave different answers, such as when the residents are all fighting, when it's bath day or when laundry arrives and when all of these things happen at one time plus a new resident comes on the unit at the same time. The one thing that is consistent across all CNAs is the mention of outsider's intrusions of one kind or another on their autonomy to provide care.

One afternoon when Marita Martin is taking a break, she talks about the CNAs' behavior and "things not getting done" when she is out sick or on vacation. She elaborates:

> Now, I know they get buried and they conduct their routines but I'm not sure little things get done like sitting with the residents, holding their hand. It's a group thing. Because there's things that should have been done that weren't being done. I give them the same speech when I come back. "Why did you allow this? You know if I was here I would have you …" And they're just like little kids, you know. No eye contact what-so-ever. And they know it. "Well, we wanted to wait until you came back," they say. The problem with other nurses coming in is that they sometimes won't go by what the CNA says. CNAs know the resident better than nurses do. It's like the stepmother comes in. It's like "My mom's gone."

Several important insights come from Marita's comments. In summoning up the "stepmother" analogy, Marita is searching for an answer. On the one hand, there may well be a reality here based on Marita's perspective; however, working within the framework of intrusions on autonomy and the concept of teamwork as an essential part of identity for the CNAs, there may be other plausible interpretations. When Marita Martin is gone, the occasion for a major threat to staff's autonomy occurs. First, teamwork and team decision-making is of utmost importance to the Alzheimer's staff. In Carma Lee's revealing metaphor, to have a member of the team absent is "Like having a finger missing." Moreover, the absence of LPN Marita becomes significant in its consequences; she is a former CNA who works at "not forgetting" her "earlier rank and its demands." Thus, one arbiter between the CNAs and the administration (the other being RN Elaine Pressley) is unavailable.

Second, Marita recognizes that "some nurses do not listen to what the CNAs say, that some of the LPNs feel like 'I'm the nurse. I'm in charge. Why do I have to listen to the CNA.'" Such a dismissal of staff knowledge can become a primary threat to the identity of the CNAs and the moment to moment exercise of their skills on their own terms. When queried as to what happens when Marita has to be on leave, the CNAs offer a slight variation on Arnella's contention that "Things don't really go well. They try to change things. It upsets us." With a hint of self-promotion while articulating her own position of strength, Marita also acknowledges the interdependency of the team and the reality of meeting the demands of her job when she says:

> You have to listen to the CNA or you're going to learn nothing because those girls have made me who I am today. I'd be lost without them. I wouldn't be known as Marita Martin, the Unit Coordinator of the Alzheimer's Pavilion. Why do they send me to seminars? Why do families come to me and tell me how much they appreciate things. It's because of the CNAs. They're my spine. Without them I can't stand up.

Three structural issues on the Pavilion provoke the staff and intrude on their autonomy. First, the timing of lunch trays with delayed sequences poses lunchtime problems for the staff because some residents are served while others have to wait. Residents without trays see others with food, which creates much agitation at the table. "Temperature regularity" (maintaining state-mandated food temperature levels to benefit the residents) ends up being a deficit for both residents and staff. Second, complications associated with the task of putting away residents' laundry becomes much more difficult in that clothes are not pre-sorted and all arrive at the same time based on institutional mandates instead of the needs of the Pavilion. Finally, Marita speaks to the issue of placement on the unit: "When they can't solve a problem like someone that's disruptive or shouting upstairs (in the nursing home) of course the solution is the Alzheimer's Pavilion. They have somewhat of a diagnosis of Alzheimer's disease." All three issues illustrate the paradox of rationalization as irrational. "It can really make you go off sometimes," Chevelle laments.

The "Courtesy Appearance"

> Sometimes I think they (families, professionals, administration) just think the girls are here to change, to sit with. I think sometimes people come down here just for show. I really hate to say that. To show they're CONcerned. And I really don't see a concern. Sometimes it just absolutely frazzles me when they (administration) come and do a courtesy appearance and that's all it is—a courtesy appearance.
>
> *Marita Martin*

When discussing a major source of their struggle, the staff identify the lack of the administration's and some families' interest and attempts at understanding the nature and demands of their "different care." Carma Lee argues,

> The administration doesn't want to understand. As long as someone is taking care of the residents that's about it. They just need to come and observe and look more regularly. Just to see what we're doing. It wouldn't have to be anything special. Just maybe twice a week to come see what goes on, how we work.

Arnella would like to have recognition and an audience for their ideas as she says:

> If they would just come and listen to us and watch us. Like I said we don't even know how far anything is goin' but I think that if Mr. Greenberg or the Board of Directors or whoever else would come and have a meeting with us and listen to some of our ideas that we have. And come and visit. We don't know who's on the Board. Come and make yourself known. We're both going only by what we hear. Let's everybody meet and know one another and know what's going on and why.

When I asked Marita Martin if she thought the administration understood the demands of their job and the design of what they have constructed as special she comments:

> Absolutely not. Absolutely not. They don't know from what's comin' in that door. They come in. They stay as long as they want. Maybe a couple of minutes. Three, maybe five minutes and then they go out the back door. They cannot imagine. They cannot imagine how stressful it can become here at times. Because I noticed today I was getting loud. And I noticed Glenda got like that and then Chevelle got like that. And I asked myself what am I doing? Why am I using my voice like this?

Justine speaks to the invisibility of administration even though the CEO says that the Pavilion is his "baby." She comments:

> I said well my goodness for this to be his baby down here, we rarely see him. You would think when he did come he would stay. He just walks through. He'll shake so-in-so's hand and that's it. Sit, have lunch with us. Eat snacks with them. Come and help serve the snacks. Let me know this is your baby because I'm going to take pride in my baby. You know what I'm saying. I'm going to be there.

Chevelle wants to see the families come and spend some time on the Pavilion. She relates that "They (families) may bring them a gift but they only stay for 15 or 20 minutes. You know, they should stay and see what's goin' on."

To a person, the CNAs want the administration and families to see, to watch and to stay long enough to get a sense of the staff's care work, the responsibilities they have. I would argue that these concerns of the staff carry a latent meaning that focuses on two things: affiliation and bearing witness to their work. The CNAs want administration and families to come and linger for a period of time—a certain duration, enough to become socialized into the care work world they have constructed. They want to be recognized in ways that provide social value to the work they are doing in its complexity and with its demands. They want to see a demonstration of concern by staying in their world, by seeing the array of skills of the staff, and by watching what happens as the day unfolds and as the weeks go by. What they want is for someone outside the Pavilion to not only make a cursory appearance but to be concerned, to *bear witness* to the lives of residents in their care and to the work of care itself. Justine speaks of life on the Pavilion as a story. This story is an ongoing construction that unfolds day to day. Staff come in and create a world separate from the outside world. Their creation is not the fantasy—the in-service is the fantasy. The CNAs challenge those in authority (administration) and those who are responsible (family) to manifest that responsibility through *bearing witness*. On the deepest level, staff are seeking a moral commitment from administration and families to be persons who exercise agency, to be more than passive observers but bear witness to the staff's skills and body of local knowledge-in-practice.

Notes

1 Findings from a study by the American Geriatrics Core Writing Group (2010: S251) bear out Elaine Pressley's perspective. Recruitment into the specialty of geriatrics is a problem. Today there is only one geriatrician per 5,000 Americans aged 65 and older with the disparity expected to worsen by 2020 in the United States. Physicians in training are reluctant to go into geriatrics because of concern that the lifestyle will be onerous and the pay too low.

2 Michel Foucault, *The Birth of the Clinic: An Archaeology of Medical Perception* (New York: Vintage, 1973), coined the term "medical gaze" that the medical profession can use to dehumanize the patient by separating the patient's body from the patient's person. In the case of some family members the gaze is used to accomplish just that: to subdue and ridicule certain residents.

3 Jürgen Habermas, *Moral Consciousness and Communicative Action* (Cambridge, MA: The MIT Press, 1991: 138).

4 Michel Foucault, *Power/Knowledge* (New York: Pantheon Books, 1980: 81).

5 Ibid., 82.

6 Pavilion staff, RN Pressley and Director of Nursing have periodic meetings with families to address the needs of their family member and construct a plan of care for the resident. CNAs rarely go to these meetings. The meetings are held outside of the Pavilion and CNAs (including Marita Martin) feel that "nothing gets done in these meetings."

7 Marita Martin tells me that in private conversations, however, some CNAs give Henrietta Stein a derogatory nickname, "dirty Hennie," because of her racist rantings.

8

LOCAL INTELLIGENCE

Bed and body duties are ending as I walk into the Pavilion this April morning. In the distance, a CNA puts on soft rock music as LPN Marita Martin drops her paperwork, comes out of the nurse's station, dances across the floor, and extends her hand to resident Elsie Kidd. "Come on Grammaw," she says, and takes Elsie to the center of the room. Elsie Kidd, a widow with grandchildren who visit regularly and are devoted to her, loves to dance and she's good, they say. CNA Glenda has moved to the center of the room and is taking people by the hand, beckoning "Boots" (Verna) to dance. "Let's shake our booties," LPN Marita calls to the group in her coy way. CNAs Justine, Arnella and Carma have gathered at the edge of the sitting room and are beginning to clap. Usually reserved, Rachel Cowen, a former homemaker, emerges from the side and sashays into the center of the room. With that, the CNAs shout "Ouuuuuueeeee, here she comes." Rachel, who has been at the Pavilion about four years, glides around the floor, her hips swaying and her delicate arms rising above her head as if she is sculpting something in the air. When speaking with me about her Mother's difficult past of divorce and deaths in the family, Rachel's daughter exclaims, "I've never seen mother dance like that before." CNA Carma Lee's comment about the residents having a "new self" comes to mind as Rachel embraces the air around her.

We begin tapping our feet and Marita glides over to new resident, Jane Bloomberg, and invites her onto the floor. Their hands meet in a circle of dance. "Look, my new friend is gonna dance with me, and look at those big earrings," Marita calls out. Jane sports a fuchsia blouse and skirt and white shoes. A beaded black purse dangles from her arm. Jane was a teacher who never married and lived with her sister until recently when she was diagnosed with dementia. Jane's sister finds it very difficult to visit; she lacks transportation and does not "know" her sister anymore nor how to talk to her, a source of much sorrow.

Several residents begin to clap while Boris Randolph watches intently. Since his hospitalization, he does not have the sprightly gait he once had. CNA Glenda reaches for Boris and Carrie Mae. Boris appears to be confused as to what to do. "Come on Boris, this is a romantic dance," Glenda says. They position themselves and Carrie Mae looks up at Boris with a glowing smile. They embrace and begin to move ever so slightly, just enough for the entire staff to break into "Awwwwwww."

CNA Marita grasps Martin Lovett's hands so they can move in place. He is beaming and arches his shoulders up and down. Martin points to the tables in the dining area and counts, "one, two, three, four," his first words in many months. Resident Harriet French ambles over to CNA Chevelle and sways back and forth. Chevelle and I move the upper part of our bodies in response to hers. She does the same thing in return and we are "speaking a language in time" with each other. Harriet reaches down and kisses Chevelle on the cheek and rubs her face on mine. She is exuberant. To the staff's surprise, Henrietta Stein parades over to Martin Lovett and pops a kiss on his forehead. In the center of the dance floor, outfitted in a black top and tights, Elsie is doing her personal ballet. The CNAs comment that her "grandkids really dress her with lots of style." Now the music bubbles with a polka. The room is alive, abundant and generative. We all move in the same sphere it seems, differences evaporated.

During these moments, life on the Pavilion is punctuated with collective expression, which helps the staff promote the emotional well-being of resident selves. Dancing becomes a form of communication, a shared language of sorts, seemingly accomplished with ease; however, in a capricious world of varying degrees of intelligibility and striking individuality, communication with, and knowledge of, the residents is never static, often fragile and, more times than not, challenging to acquire and apply. As CNA Chevelle claims, "You have to be thinking all the time. Where's your brain now? You just never know what to expect from each one (resident)."

In the lifeworld of the Pavilion, the mundane and the extraordinary are forever in a welter of movement where a distinct buzz churns just beneath it all as ladies on sofas chatter the morning away and men with bent heads and chins on their chests, nap; where residents stand on tiptoe at the nurse's alcove to watch the head nurse record each of their waking hours devoid of the inscription of *life* in those same hours. In this world, staff weave a tapestry of knowledge on which an intricate pattern arises as they build and revise their understanding of the residents. This tapestry is an oral knowledge, which informs the operation of the Pavilion and the world within. Many times, when trying to articulate their special skills and knowledge, staff members will say, with mounting frustration, "I just can't put it into words." "I just can't find the words for what I am trying to describe." Marita Martin puts it this way:

> When I enter the Pavilion, I have to leave my normal self behind. You have to have what I call a "seventh sense" that is necessary to work on the Pavilion.

> But I can't put it into other words. Not everybody has it and I'm talking about every area of departments. You have to have the seventh sense to work on the Alzheimer's unit. If you don't have it you might as well just forget it—go work someplace else. You have to understand the capacity of the disease.

After several months on the Alzheimer's Pavilion, I began to sense a rhythm to the flow of bed and body work, rituals and collective expression. Later, Justine Jackson used the word rhythm to describe the way that she and other CNAs work as a team and care for residents amid erratic "atmospheres" and behaviors. "It's so hard to put into words. I don't know …" she says.

From another perspective, what CNAs and Marita Martin have constructed and experience as a knowledge that *defies* words may be understood on a deeper level as the epitome of *Metis*. *Metis* originates from classical Greek and designates knowledge that is derived exclusively from practice "… in contrast to formal, deductive, epistemic knowledge."[1] Detienne and Vernant[2] elucidate the concept of *metis:*

> Although *metis* … holds such an important position within the Greek system of values, it is never made manifest for what it is, it is never clearly revealed in a theoretical work that aims to define it. *Metis* is a type of wily intelligence and of thought, a way of knowing; it implies a complex but very coherent body of mental attitudes and behavior which combine flair, wisdom, forethought, subtlety of mind deception, resourcefulness, vigilance, opportunism, various skills, and experience acquired over the years. *It is applied to situations which are transient, shifting, disconcerting and ambiguous, situations which do not lend themselves to precise measurement, exact calculation or rigorous logic* (emphases are the author's).

The one constant in the staff members' daily work is unpredictability; the staff must *begin* each day facing ever-changing situations.

In *Seeing Like a State*, James Scott[3] provides additional insight into such knowledge:

> Local knowledge is as economical and accurate as it needs to be, no more and no less, for addressing the problem at hand. To begin with, skills that require adaptation to a capricious physical environment, the acquired knowledge of how to sail, fly a kite, fish, etc. rely on the capacity for *metis*. Each of these skills requires hand-eye coordination that comes with practice and a capacity to read the winds, the waves or the road and make appropriate adjustments. One powerful indication that they all require *metis* is that they are exceptionally difficult to teach apart from engaging in the activity itself … Trades requiring a touch or feel for implements and materials or in the case of human work, for the touch or feel of human needs, and circumstances require a touch and a feel. *Metis* equally applies to human

> interaction. Think of the complex physical activities that require constant adjustment to the movement, desires, or gestures of others.

In this last chapter, we focus on two major facets of the staff's different knowledge, "Tacit Knowing" and "Vigilant Eyes, Ears, and Mind" as *Metis* knowledge.

Tacit Knowing

All is quiet at 1:45 pm when LPN Marita Martin brings her paperwork over to the couch to sit among the residents. At that moment, Harriet French charges across the room, stops and faces Ruby Jacobs with a smile, extends her arm and slaps Ruby in the face. There is a murmur among the residents in close range as Marita rushes across the room to intercept Harriet before she strikes again. A palpable tension arises with several residents glaring at Harriet and looking at each other. LPN Marita comments on her approach to Harriet:

> I was upset with her. I know lots of times when I want to express control with them I will grab 'em from their wrist and I'll look directly in their eyes and let them see through my windows how I feel about it. She was ok after. I don't like this thing of hitting people. See she did this before when she first came here. She beat the heck out of us if we wanted to dress her, to change her and then she became incontinent and then it became even worse. Then they took her off the medication, some kind of anticonvulsant. The daughter said she had seizures but we never saw any seizures from day one.

Marita sensed an "aura" on the Pavilion, as she has a number of times before. Recognizing auras serves a large purpose for Marita—anticipation and control of disruptive behavior that can escalate to other residents. Through experience, she knows something without being able to explain *how* she knows it. She arrives at this tacit knowledge "… through internal reflection."[4]

Efforts at communication in ordinary discourse among individuals without cognitive deficits can be laden with numerous possibilities for misinterpretation and misunderstanding. At Starrmount, the challenge of verbal communication with Alzheimer's residents can be formidable. Awareness of residents' varying states of being test the mettle of staff. CNAs speak about being able to "sense" various states of mind, attitudes, and feelings of the residents. When trying to give words to a phenomenon which they have never sought to articulate because it has never been put to them, staff remark with a sense of confidence, "We know … just know." Theirs is an almost instantaneous understanding that provides one form of communication despite the looming presence of changing intelligibility among the residents. Justine grapples with putting this into words:

> Just because they (the residents) don't follow directions or you have to feed them, it doesn't mean they don't understand. There's still something there that they can pick up. You don't know. Something might spark a memory. We all feel the same way. We were talking about this not too long ago that isn't it strange how we know. But I told them that that's innate. For some reason we just know. We just know what they're asking. We know.

"Just knowing" is a result of a lot of hard work over several years, nourished and shared by the group. Justine suggests that tacit knowledge is a part of each staff member. The exclusive nature of this knowledge is implied in Justine's remark that a tacit knowing capacity is "innate." At the same time, it is important to remember that we have seen where blatant racism and intrusions on CNAs' autonomy from family, medicine and administration can elicit reactivity, anger and defensive behavior on the part of staff.

An excerpt from field notes of my trying to help resident Bertha Waker move from the family room to the dining table provides a glimpse into the demands of a particular kind of "knowing" through touch and strength:

> The call and gathering for breakfast has pretty much ended with two or three residents lingering in the sitting room. Resident Ellen Draper is standing in front of me and I ask her if she would like to have breakfast. She smiles and nods her head. I take her by the arm and walk her over to the far table where she slips into her seat. I return to the sitting room to fetch frail and partially blind Bertha Waker. With as much care and strength as I can muster, I am able to get her up from her seated position and steady her on her feet. We creep toward the table and she looks up at me and says, "God bless you." Chevelle looks at us with a smile and says, "Bertha, you're walking real good." We arrive at the table and it dawns on me that Bertha can't see and I will need to guide her gingerly into the chair. She is so grateful when she squeezes my hand. As I lower her into the seat, I realize what a responsibility all of this is and how much sheer physical strength, to say nothing of the mental strength it takes to work on this Pavilion.

All CNAs and Marita Martin contend that expenditure of mental energy far outweighs the physical. Physical touch and tone of voice are crucial as a means of bringing about change in resident behavior. The "morning approach" to a resident can have a significant effect on the emotional tenor of a resident's entire day.

"Reading of Physiognomy"

We are seated in the back parlor of the Alzheimer's Pavilion in front of the large glass windows. Paths of glistening water inch down the glass as the rain pelts down in the courtyard. My mind wanders for a moment as I ponder the contrasts of "inching" and "pelting" as metaphorically speaking about the contrast of whole lives lived in the rhythm of the Pavilion world in comparison with the frantic rhythms of outside society. I slide back into focus as Marita Martin speaks and notice out of the corner of my eye that Boris Randolph is ambling over to us. He stops next to me, dressed in hat, shirt, sports jacket and dress pants. His hands are in his pockets and he has a wry smile on his face with a bit of a furrowed brow:

ANNE: Greetings. You seem very active this afternoon.
BORIS: (his blue eyes looking directly into mine) Well, I got in from the line. I was just trying to think what they are …
ANNE: (smiling playfully) Are you trying to decide what to do?
BORIS: Uh huh … Bunch of people back there you know (said in an official tone).
MARITA: (whispering, darting her eyes to mine and translating) Change of shifts.
ANNE: Well, can I catch ya later?
BORIS: Ok. I'll take another look.
MARITA: (turning to me) What did he just tell us?
ANNE: What comes to your mind?
MARITA: There's lots of people back there (in the nurse's station). He's talking about the change of shifts. It confuses him sometimes because he doesn't understand why everybody's back there. He's more comfortable when they go out and sit with them (the residents) than he is with them all in the back. But realize that he was the comptroller of a bank. Sometimes that window (around the nurse's station) reminds him and he thinks that money's back there. That's what I think. He's concerned.

It is common for certain residents to seek out pockets of interaction on the Pavilion and to drift into the "goings on" among staff, or between the staff and me. In this example, Marita Martin utilizes a prime opportunity to demonstrate and affirm her skills to me. Her question serves as a quiz to one who is not privy to different knowledge. Her explanation is an example of the interpretive and interactive aspect of an ongoing investigative process.

One of the ways staff read residents' wants and needs is akin to a "reading of physiognomy." In understanding the mood of a person, for example worry, Polanyi[5] states that we note the

> furrowed brow, the downcast eyes, the lowered body, the heaviness of movement, the pinched voice and mouth, and other clues in catching the whole mood … Together they enable a reading of the person's state of being or mental outlook.

A reading of physiognomy for the staff involves a concentration on "signs," gestures, and body language of the resident, as CNA Carma Lee explains:

> You have to anticipate what they need down here. Being with them so many hours out of the year, you know them. You know what they need. Are they in pain? Do they have a headache? How do we know these things? We tell Marita, "Well you know they don't look right. Look at their eyes and look at the way they look. Look at their face."

"Reading" may involve detecting physical needs such as wanting to go to the bathroom. Arnella comments:

> First of all, we use a lot of … (pausing), I can't really say sign language, but you have to do a lot of watching. Most of the time I can look at a person and tell if something is bothering them. Like they may be in distress. They may not say anything to you, but just in watching you can see. You hear a lot just by observing. Like for instance, Elise. She's constantly walking around with her eyes closed and we have to call to her to open them. I can usually tell when she has to go to the bathroom because her face will get tight, tight around the mouth instead of calm while she's walking around.

Arnella expresses a capacity for tacit knowing in terms of what might be bothering a resident. She considers her "reading" capability to be an asset in her work. Whether or not she intended to say, "You hear (auditory) a lot just by observing" (visual), it is interesting to speculate on the multiple senses employed in her care work. The skill of being able to "read" human interaction, in the sense Arnella and the CNAs are speaking of, is a complex skill that requires constant adjustment to the movement, values, desires or gestures of others.

Arnella drives home the importance of work experience on the Pavilion. Implicit in her comments is the prior accumulation of tacit knowledge that is employed to "anticipate" what residents need, or try to predict what might happen given present behavior. She suggests that reading of body signs from the staff's perspective can have two major outcomes: first, as an end in itself where the staff know and identify the need and are able to meet it; and second, as a prelude to their calling in the physician to take a look at the resident. Marita told me that she thinks "the girls are experts at this knowing and have taught me about it."

Employing tacit knowledge can extend to a family member visiting on the Pavilion. CNA Arnella "reads" countenance and draws implications in describing a poignant greeting between a son and his mother on the Pavilion. She relates:

> ARNELLA: Basically, Simon asks how his mother is doing. If she needs anything. He really doesn't talk a lot…about…his…mother, because it bothers him and I know it does.

ANNE: How do you know?

ARNELLA: Well, when he comes in and like if he catches Mary Louise's eye and Elise smiles at him, he'll smile back. He's got grief written all over his face. I mean it's sad. Especially if he goes over and he might hug her and then Mary may say something that doesn't totally make sense to him and I know it gets to him (a forlorn quality in Arnella's voice).

Arnella's tacit knowing is noteworthy for her grasp of the delicate chords of response between Simon Cutler and his mother, Mary Louise, a woman of stately bearing and grace. In the three-hour interview that I spent with Simon and his wife in my home, I came to understand the distant relationship between mother and son. Today the relationship is growing because of the lack of inhibition in his mother and in himself; however, it is also laden with the ever-present sadness of the lost woman–mother, the once elegant, fastidious wife of a prominent man. These are the facts of Simon's life as expressed in the interview with me, something Arnella would not know in the sense of social facts. Yet, she grasped, in a tacit sense, the essence of the relating, even down to pointing out, what can be viewed as the "silent communication" from across the room when a son comes seeking his mother.

Vigilant Eyes, Ears and Mind

One morning, Marita Martin and I are deep in conversation. She tells me, "I'm a gad-about and I love to meet people, talk to people from different cultures. I get excited about the simplest things and want to—." Abruptly, she stops in mid-sentence and turns her head to the opposite corner of the sitting room. "Excuse me, I don't think I've ever heard her talk that much. It's moments like this that we need to be there." Marita is referring to the sustained conversation between two residents. She notes:

> The two of them are sitting on the couch not only absorbed in conversation but turn-taking. See, everybody thinks I'm just sitting back there writing but I have big ears. I hear everything. I hear everything that goes on, even some of the stuff that is commented on over there (pointing to the dining area). See, I don't let anybody know that. Like when I'm sitting at the desk and they're around the corner at the dinette, conversations or comments are made. I hear them.

Prior to a first interview with the CNAs and LPN Marita Martin, I recorded in my field notes what appeared to be an uncommon capacity for, and practice of, intense watching.

One day a staff member summed up the watching phenomenon when she posed a question and answered it: "How many eyes and ears does one need to work in this place? Thousands."

Purposeful Watchfulness

LPN Marita keeps a notebook (separate from chart entries) on the behavior of residents, down to the smallest details. These notes have two purposes. First, they are aimed at capturing present behavior, changes in behavior, and anticipating what might be coming to strategize with the CNAs on how best to control destructive behavior in a dynamic environment. Second, for Marita as well as the CNAs, purposeful watching looks to improving strategies for activating a resident's "mind" and giving emotional support. Marita confided that she sometimes takes notes on residents to ponder at home. On several occasions, I witnessed Marita's watching as though there was a churning field of energy going on within her head that matched the energy outside it.

The first day that a new resident enters the Pavilion, CNAs Arnella, Carma Lee, Justine and Chevelle will adjust their schedules to allow for informal concentration on the resident's habits and preferences. Beginning during this time, the apprenticeship to the new Alzheimer's resident varies in intensity from aide to aide, and involves a certain protocol. Arnella explains:

> We greet the resident and the family. Take them to their room. While we're talking, while Marita is assessing the resident, we're listening to what the residents say. Then we basically look them over from head to toe. Make sure there are no scratches on them, cuts, bruises. We chart down what we find. We do an inventory of their clothing and other property. We count it. We describe it. We put all that down on paper. That goes in the chart. But we *listen* to what the residents say. The *tone*. The tone of voice. We're looking at facial expressions, body *gestures*.

Arnella makes it clear that the very first observational interest is on the body, the physicality of the self; however, the significant word in Arnella's narrative is "but," signaling, through intonation, an important delineation about to come. She distinguishes an objectification of a new resident imposed by institutional regulations and medical necessity from what she implies is the real task: listening and looking with resourcefulness for the subtle and revealing aspects of the person in their midst. As Arnella puts it, listening and looking for a person's "*tone*."

On one level, Arnella's description is an example of competent CNAs carrying out their duties of obtaining medical information as part of the routine entrance examination onto the Pavilion. On another level, it is an example of how selective recording in the chart imposed by the institution can force a circumscribed identity on the resident, eliminating the CNA's totality of care. Arnella counters this by turning it on its head as she discursively reconstructs the meaning of "charting down" in contrast to "listening to" and observing the "tone" of the resident. She counters the institutional meaning through her latent meaning: the chart as incomplete record, as though the real, most important things are saved for the CNAs' heads.

As time moves on, initial observation of the resident gives way to what can be called "purposeful watchfulness." Observation is prompted by a new resident coming on the Pavilion or sometimes by special events such as physical sickness, and precipitous behavior changes. There is a qualitative distinction between purposeful watching and observation. Purposeful watchfulness is the *ongoing* effort to understand individual residents, and create meaning out of an array of vivid behaviors, moods and competencies. Watching denotes monitoring the residents to handle potential behavioral problems; however, staff replace the objectifying "gaze" with the goal of comprehending the resident, seeing and understanding, in the words of CNA Glenda Morgan, "what irritates them, what calms them down, what makes them laugh." In the following exchange, Carma and Arnella talk about Martin Lovett, the 79-year-old former television news anchor who never speaks except for reading out loud:

CARMA: Martin likes to read a lot. I watch him.

ANNE: (in a surprised tone) Does he still read? What does he read?

ARNELLA: Well, like, say for instance there's a piece of paper on the bulletin board. He'll go over to the bulletin board and he will read it.

CARMA: And he reads it aloud.

ANNE: And you've been around when he has done this and he will read the words as they are?

ARNELLA: Uh Huh. He'll come around the desk and the menu is up on the glass and he'll read it.

CARMA: Or he'll read the calendar. He'll quote what today is.

I am surprised by what Carma Lee means by "read." I have an image of Martin Lovett sitting and reading a book, magazine or newspaper; both CNAs mean something different. I am constructing a meaning to her comments situated in what I carry around as the dominant culture's definition of reading. CNAs are constructing meaning from the context of "local culture" where reading, among other things, takes on alternative meanings. Through their purposeful watching, Carma Lee and Arnella understand that Martin Lovett only speaks out loud when he reads public announcements because such behavior is tied to his past occupation. Mr. Lovett was a "reader of the news" as an anchorman on television for many years. Arnella emphasizes that,

> You can't treat all of them alike. Some of them you have to treat with kid gloves. You get better results, you know, when you're gentle with them. If you come to them real aggressive then all you'll get is resistance.

The watching phenomenon extended to me when I first came to the Pavilion. After I had been there for about six months, Justine revealed that the CNAs had been watching me for a long time because "We wanted to see how you treated the residents." Of course, I had the same intention in my observation of them. When a level of trust was established between the staff and me, watching served another purpose: assisting me as a participant observer on the Pavilion. In the following, I get CNAs' assistance as well as humorous direction from resident Marge Jacobs, as both parties are watching me from a distance:

> Resident Ruth Dixon is eating ice cream and has dropped the cookie with the ice cream on her leg but doesn't seem to notice. I try to point it out but she doesn't understand. I look for a tissue. The aides are aware of my search and point to a bathroom where I can get a paper towel. I bring it back and clean up Ruth. CNA Diane is also watching and she points to the trashcan down the corridor for me to deposit the soiled paper towel. I ask Ruth to give me the newspaper in which she has wrapped the "bib" but she is reluctant. I try again and ask, "May I take this, please let me take this and you can keep the bib." With that, resident Marge Jacobs interrupts her chanting, "1, 2, 3, Out Goes She into the deep blue"—to say to me in an exasperated manner, "Yes go ahead and take it, for pete's sake just *take* it …" Laughter overtakes us all.

Feminist scholar and poet, Audre Lorde, comments that

> In order to survive, those of us for whom oppression is as American as apple pie have always had to be "watchers," to become familiar with the language and manners of the oppressor, even sometimes adopting them for some illusion of protection.[6]

As "watchers," the staff take that developed capacity and turn it into a critical skill.

Discovery Work

> *Metis* resists simplification into deductive principles … because the environments in which it is exercised are so complex and non-repeatable that formal procedures of rational decision making are impossible to apply. In a sense, *metis* lies in that large space between the realm of genius, to which no formula can apply, and the realm of codified knowledge, which can be learned by rote.
>
> —*James Scott*[7]

At this early morning hour, a downpour makes the view into the courtyard a collection of watery images. Still, Miss Ava Reynolds presses her nose against the glass to look out, her miniature pigtail adorned with an equally miniature, crisply tied white ribbon. CNA Justine must have had her in the nurse's station doing her hair and nails earlier today, a Friday morning tradition. Miss Ava becomes a center of attention on these days. RN Elaine Pressley says, "The staff do have their favorites." Miss Ava turns and sees me coming. "Oh now, don't you look ba-a-ad this mornin', you lookin' so cute. Just as bad as you can be," she says. "Well, you're lookin' baad yourself, Miss Ava," I say, and give her a hug on my way to meet Justine Jackson to continue our conversation from yesterday.

CNA Justine relates several instances of discovery work in which she displays elements of developing hunches, and gathering evidence through watching, reflecting, and developing a hypothesis to be verified over time. The first example shows the duration of her watching with 83-year-old resident, Ava Reynolds, one of two Black residents. The staff say that Justine is the only one who can "do anything" with Miss Ava when she gets "agitated." Justine has been told that Miss Ava was initiating fights with other residents, an evaluation Justine cannot accept. Justine explains her reasoning:

> I had to really watch because they said Ava was picking fights. I said, "I just don't believe it" (very animated). And I watched and when she's in that room, Ava usually has everything spread out and everything. Don't bother it. Don't go in there. Don't bother anything. If you do you're messing with her things. I learned that from experience. I had to watch her. It took me about six months to really learn this, but I did. Then I told everybody else. She's not going to bother anybody. If she hits somebody, it's because they are doing something to her. It may be that person's property that Ava has but they can't just go and say give me that. That's mine. No, they're going to get slapped upside the head.

Justine's commitment to the process of discovery work in knowledge gathering is implicit in this quote and explicit in the length of time that she has watched. What could appear as *un*-reasonable behavior becomes, according to Justine's investigation and construction, behavior *with*-reason. Accurate knowledge about an incident is crucial to maintaining the integrity of, and exercising responsibility for, the persisting self of the resident. Simultaneously, getting to the bottom of potentially disruptive behavior adds to the CNA's skills to foresee trouble when others infringe on Aunt Ava's "territory."

Further confirmation of Justine's hypothesis was accomplished through collecting evidence when Miss Ava moved to share a room with another resident:

> Ava got into it with Florence. Florence had been in that room so long by herself, that it was hers. When Ava came, Florence would wait until Ava laid down and pour water on her. So, Ava got up and hit her. We watched Ava for a couple of months and (verifying) unless you really do something to her you, you have to mess with her before she … other than that she'll sit quietly. Leave her alone and she won't bother you. And she can be a lot of

> fun. She's a real pleasant lady. She has a dirty mouth if you make her mad. She can be a lot of fun to talk to. She likes to laugh.

On these two occasions, the check mark in the official resident chart may read "agitated" for Ava Reynolds because the domination of the medical model eliminates alternative choices to capture *on paper* the true nature of the incident. The staff's discovery work and knowledge is not given *language* in the official chart. Within the chart, Miss Ava is not read as a person (a self) but as a bundle of symptoms and vital signs at worst or as dependent at best. But, *here is the form of resistance: it stays in the heads of the CNAs* and becomes a part of the script, or "story" of the construction of care that is the antithesis of a rationalized model. Both instances involve the possibility of negative labeling of Aunt Ava as the culprit, had Justine not investigated.

A learning process, discovery work can best be termed an informal *apprenticeship* to the Starrmount Alzheimer's residents, which focuses on finding meaning in resident actions and attempting to *foresee* future resident behavior that can be disruptive. CNA Chevelle reflects on her approach in the following passage:

> Learning, I think is basically it. Some of them a noise irritates them, and you just take them off and just talk quietly. And some of the answers that they give you when I'm talking to them one on one fascinates me. I learned from them actually. I really did. To me, it's the same as going to school, your math and stuff you have to read. I sit back and I watch ("read") them, their actions, how they act toward different things. And learn from them, what irritates them, what calms them down, what makes them laugh. They even taught me some subjects you can talk to them about. They're really, really serious. They really get with you, and sometimes I have to jump right in there with them and learn from the residents. When they first come in we have to watch them, *learn them for ourselves.*

In Chevelle's analogy to "going to school" there is the implicit idea of a *method* to the process which is cumulative in nature, shaped and directed by the diversity and individuality of the residents, and the capabilities and awareness of the aides. Embedded in this comment, and supported by months of observation at Starrmount, there is a learning from and a learning about diverse subjects through the residents' recollections. Such subjects may range from science, a typology of trees from former resident, Doc. Smith, to food (secrets of making pumpkin pie from 74-year-old Sara Gordon, a former housewife, mother of three, whose husband is deceased), to philosophy on early childhood rearing from Fay Morgan (an 82-year-old mother of twin boys of whom she is most proud). In the telling, residents allow glimpses into their identities, past and present. Some staff do not want second-hand knowledge of the residents, nor to know what they did before coming to Starrmount, except as it may emerge from the resident. While Chevelle wants to know from the family about activities and interests of the resident, she is reluctant to accept characterizations of the resident's personality, temperament and idiosyncrasies.

Using the metaphor of learning subjects in school, Chevelle casts the residents in the role of teacher, a generative elder. The resident has passed something old on to Chevelle, which she experiences as "fascinating." RN Elaine Pressley captures the sentiment well when she says, "You know, I'd love to look into some of their brains. Henrietta Stein for example. I would love to know what makes her tick. To me, she's intriguing."

Discovery work is stimulated at times by the complexity of the disease and associated behavior to just figure it out, and by the need to control behavior. Much of the time, staff seek greater knowledge of how to provide emotional support to the resident struggling through the assaults of dementia. With a combination of thought and feeling, Charge Nurse Marita seeks answers as to why residents come to her as she sits doing paperwork in the nursing station. The station is accessible to the residents through two small, swinging doors. The partition-like sides that encase it have see-through plastic in the top half to allow residents visual access to the CNAs and the goings on in the small space. Marita asks,

> Why do they come to us? Why do they look to me and they do look to me. I'm proud of this because I must be doing something but my focus isn't quite right yet. Do they come to me because they were denied something? Is it because somebody was harsh with them? Is it because they want to be around me? What is it? I haven't come to that conclusion yet. I'm still working on it. Louisa is the one who always comes back here. Her and Carrie Mae.

Marita poses questions which center on the affective and psychological dimensions of the person with the disease as well as the person giving the care. There are questions that must be answered if only she had time to devote to study what she gathers.

Arnella talks about refining her approach to discovery work:

> First of all, you need to learn the person's habits. Be able to be a problem solver. I mean you have to know when not to push them. Try not to be tense around them because they will pick up on that and don't show your fear because that's a big mistake. Some of the little people down here, they like to hit you like Harriet. She doesn't give any warning. She may just sneak up on you and hit you in the back and keep going. If they know you're scared they'll do that to get you and you won't be able to get anything out of them.

CNA Arnella's narrative reveals an observational method, sensitivity to temporality, a use of reflexivity for her own protection from residents who excel in unpredictable behavior of a combative nature.

The following examples reveal the intricacy of two important purposes of CNA discovery work, which can occur simultaneously. In the first example, Arnella relates an experience that displays the tenterhooks on which CNAs stand when caring for and engaging Harriet French:

> I was trying to change her blouse—she had spilled some food on her blouse and I was trying to change it. She had something in her hand and she kept shaking it up in my face and I kept moving back and I said, "Now come on Harriet. Let me change your blouse," and she started fussing with me. I said, "come on now, Harriet. All I want to do is change your blouse." She just kept going on and on and I said, "Well, since you want to fight I'm just going to leave you alone then." She could tell by the tone of my voice that I was scared. I didn't know if she was going to hit me or what. I must have looked up or something because she kicked me in my leg and from then on I knew even if I was scared or fearful of what she might do I couldn't let her know that.

A skill that the staff employ when a strategy is not working is to retreat and come back to the resident later. Arnella describes how she learned to "mask" her emotions when getting Harriet French to do what she wants her to do. Implicit in this encounter, is a contest of power. Arnella names her own emotion and the unpredictability of the moment in response to Harriet French. Arnella "knows" that Harriet could "tell by the tone in my voice that I was scared." She attributes to a resident the capacity for tacit knowing, which creates an instant of equalizing power between caregiver and resident. Arnella blames a lapse in her own watching ("I must have looked up") for a power shift favoring Harriet French who kicked her in the leg.

The second example of the different purposes toward which care work is directed concerns the CNAs' attention to identifying and facilitating behavior that "triggers" what they hypothesize is a pleasurable memory for the residents. Skills such as this provide emotional support, calm the resident, and require keen watching over time on the part of the staff. Marita Martin explains:

> You look at them while they are eating and they're like, "Boy, this really tastes good." And you look at them and you want to keep that every day. You want to keep them at that level. If they do this every single day the same way it's going to trigger something. Not everybody understands what we are talking about now. Or even to brush their hair all the time. Mildred Summers, she's stopped. She used to love to brush her hair. It's nice and thick. She'd brush her hair and brush her hair and she used to get such enjoyment out of that brush. So make sure that she has that brush. She'd sit there for hours just brushing that hair and she wouldn't let that brush down for anything. She would carry it around with her. To her, this is enjoyment

> and you wonder what is it about her stroking her scalp that feels so good? What is it? I've had so many questions that have been unanswered. You wouldn't believe! I can't find my paper with all of this moving around but I carry a tablet of big questions to myself—why? Yes, I brush my hair and it feels good but I don't enjoy it as much as she did. What does that bring back to her? When she was a child, did her mom stroke her head? Maybe it's related to an embrace but it has to be related to a touch.

Discovery work for CNA Glenda combines "paying close attention" to hostility between residents and purposeful watching over time to figure out how to resolve the problem if possible. She relates what she discovered as a clue that a resident was ready to "blow up" at the dining table:

> Sometimes at lunch, Henrietta keeps repeating, "I'm hungry, I'm hungry, hungry. Bring me my food!" Right after that Emily will get so mad and start screaming. Seemed like those two things were connected but I didn't know how because sometimes Emily had no reaction and things were peaceful. So I kept watchin' for a long, long time and find out that when Emily whispers to herself and it builds up, she will start screaming. So I can get in there early and stop her before she starts screaming. It's worked several times for me when I hear Emily start to whisper, "Shut up you crazy thing. She's a nut." Then I'll say, "Emily don't pay any attention. Don't let her upset you. She'll calm down."

Glenda tracks "whispering" as a sign of *impending* disturbance which not only affects those directly involved but reverberates among all residents at the dining table and brings on collective distress.

CNA Carma Lee Nelson is particularly interested in what she refers to as the "self-esteem" of the residents. Her discovery work tends to gravitate toward uncovering "self-issues" of the resident:

> Let's take Ruby for instance. She's a type of lady that she likes to have a *lot of self*, because some days she'll have, oh, you might say a blue day. Like yesterday was a bad day for her. She needs a lot of encouragement that "you're so pretty. Oh, Ruby, you're so pretty. Let's put on makeup. Let's do this, let's do that. Ben's coming, and they still love you." Basically, just listening to her over a period of months when she's whimpering, asking questions. I've found out that listening and asking questions are the best ways for me to find out what a patient needs, if they can communicate. You find a lot out by just listening because she'll tell you that she feels awful. "I wish I were dead."

The emotional reassurance offered by Carma is directly tied to what the CNAs have determined are vital sources of selfhood to Ruby Jacobs, her habit of dress and her appearance in public, thus the nickname Miss Vogue. Carma Lee's phrase, "needs a lot of self," calls forth a vivid image in contrast to Ruby's small, frail stature. Carma Lee speaks of a "blue day" for Ruby, which she understands from her own life.

Discovery work for CNA Arnella has led to her cultivation of a skill that recognizes there may be *multiple* meanings of the behavior of a resident that she needs to ponder in her care work. She elaborates:

> Sometimes with Harriet, if she's real agitated it might not be that she's upset with anybody. She may be trying to tell us that she just wants somebody to talk to her. Maybe hug her or hold her hand or something. It may not be that someone always did something to her. She may feel that she is not getting enough attention at the time. Things can have several meanings with one resident.

CNAs learn that premature closure on interpreting behavior impedes care work and they must listen and look for alternative interpretations.

Staff make a distinction between what they interpret as intentional behavior on the part of residents and behavior driven by the disease process which they see as unintentional. Attributing intentionality can direct the interaction between CNA and resident. For example, when Arnella is kicked by resident Harriet French she frames a question that, out of frustration and anger, looks for logic in the behavior:

> One time after she kicked me I asked Harriet, "Why did you do that? Have I done something to you?" She just shakes her head no. Are you sure? What would make you kick somebody? She just stands and stares at me. I would just like to know why, really.

In looking for logic in the kicking incident, Arnella attributes reasoned forethought to Harriet. Arnella's care approach to Harriet is predicated on a belief that what Harriet does (hitting) is intentional. Therefore, Arnella is tempted, in spite of herself, to elicit a reason from Harriet not only to defend herself but to discover an explanation that might allow her to repair a slight and make sense of the behavior. Making a "breakthrough" would bring about a resolution. What Arnella is left with, however, is more frustration.

Marita Martin shares Arnella's view of intentionality on the part of Harriet French of whom she says, "Harriet, I think sometimes studies before she does it like should I do this or not? There's intention. That's what I've noticed about her. She stands there and it's like she is thinkin' about doing somethin' premeditated." In fact, Marita takes Harriet's intentionality a step further in her use of "premeditated" if one thinks of premeditation as "thought-out" or "studied." She attributes a kind of complex thinking to resident self. One strategy that Carma Lee uses to lessen stress is "to visualize what it must be like for them and put myself in their place and picture myself being in that situation and that they're sick and it's part of the sickness." That, of course, does not always work.

Other cases of attributing intentionality to residents concern Henrietta Stein and Alice Caar. At an early morning staff meeting, CNAs complain about "the trails of diarrhea" that Hennie has in the mornings leading from her room to the public sitting room and back. "I think she does it on purpose, I really do," one CNA comments and the others appear to agree. While they are on the topic of excrement in unusual places, Justine comments that she thinks that "Alice Caar just knows what she is doing when she hides all those colostomy bags behind the register in her room. We go behind there and keep finding them." Justine told me in one of her interviews that "it just makes me angry and I have to settle myself in the 'cooler' for a little while."

In a last example of trying to understand likely acts of intentionality, Chevelle tries to figure out why a resident is hitting her and arrives at a reason-based explanation. She considers several possibilities including one predicated on intentionality, racism:

> Like, why are these people beating me? Is it color? Is it something else? There's something that's kicking them off. Mary Louise will hurt you. She's strong for one thing. I can get angry, you have to deal with a lot. You can't be screaming and hollering with these people. You can't do that.

While Chevelle probes why she is being hit and questions if race could be the reason, Glenda is sure that Henrietta Stein's blatant racist behavior is intentional: "We say, 'No Hennie, you can't have coffee, doctor's orders.' She calls us the n-word for saying that." The repetitive nature of Henrietta Stein's demands mixed with her intelligence and a kind of fearlessness is a formidable challenge.

Employing Wily Intelligence: "Our Own Little Language"

One afternoon, I notice that Marita has a roving eye that moves slowly over the lower extremities of residents in the sitting room. She lingers for a moment on each of the residents as though assessing something and makes notes on a manila pad. Curious, I ask her to explain. She relates something she hasn't told anyone about (even Elaine Pressley), her scale of "one to ten":

> Tedhose are white socks that people who have edema of the lower extremities wear for support. I'm looking around and they all know me. They all know what I'm thinking because I'm looking at legs. I'm looking at shoes, who has shoes on, who doesn't have shoes on. Because I like to keep a list of, in the behavior that I try to study myself, what level of Alzheimer's are they in on a scale of one to ten when they start not wanting to wear their shoes,

> or when they take their shoes off, put them back on, put the socks on, take off the socks. There's a thing about shoes.

LPN Marita speaks of "levels" of change in residents and locating them on her scale of "one to ten" to evaluate their functioning. In their social construction of alternative care, staff have developed what they call their "own little language" in which they assign alternative meanings to extant terms and concepts, and create new ones. A major way that social meanings are constructed in the Pavilion is through language in what I call a "naming and reframing" process. This process involves a reshaping of prevailing concepts from indigenous knowledge, experience and the empirical world.

The language in use in the social world of the Alzheimer's Pavilion is a distinct counterpoint to what I term a medical "language of limits," which restricts language to the realm of medical concerns and excludes the experiential and interpersonal context of the patient. In contrast, a "language of openings" is part of the staff's way of operating that focuses on the self and lifeworld of the residents, thereby honoring context. A contrast between the "medical language of limits" and a "language of openings" is a contrast in the way reality is mediated to individuals. As such, naming and reframing have two very important implications for the operation of the Alzheimer's Pavilion and the assumptions upon which it is built. First, it alters the *referent*, from the disease or biological symptoms to the person of the resident, from the behavior to the person *with* the behavior. Second, it alters the context, from the abstract medical theory and language to the *lived* context of the Alzheimer's Pavilion. In the naming and reframing process, the self of the resident has a measure of agency. Reframing constructs a set of social meanings that depict the resident as a responsive actor with some dimensions of a surviving self that is living and not just waiting to die.

Wandering versus "Getting Busy," "Moving," and "Walking"

Staff refer to persons under their care as residents rather than patients. When one is labeled as a patient and begins to behave like one, certain symptoms that may have been transient become "locked in" as appropriate or associated with the role of patient.[8] The label has been accomplished. A classic example of this in the medical literature is the "wandering" phenomenon of "unpredictable pacing without a goal" associated with Alzheimer's disease as an accompanying indicator and outcome of the disease. Lyman[9] observes that "the relativity of this definition becomes clear if it is applied to a young man pacing the halls of a maternity ward." Members of the staff suggest that there are alternative meanings to continual "movement" by Alzheimer's residents (defined as "wandering" in the medical model, which connotes aimless, meaningless movement). Only once did any staff member use the word wandering in interviews. Furthermore, I never heard it used during my months of observation on the Pavilion. Rather, CNAs speak of residents "stirring," "moving," "movin' on," "keepin' busy," "walking," "pacing," or "staying busy"—words connoting or connected with some purpose. This alternative language depicts a social world where resident's movements are treated as having meaning, a puzzle to solve or unknowable.

Confabulation versus "Going from Drive to Reverse"

When looking at the residents' charts, one often notes the sentence, "The patient was using confabulation in conversation." Confabulation can be defined medically[10] in the following way:

> The unconscious filling in of gaps of memory with fabricated facts and experiences, commonly seen in organic amnestic syndrome. It differs from lying in that the patient has no intention to deceive and believes the fabricated memories to be real.

Medical usage has taken a word without an evaluative connotation and given it one. According to the Oxford English Dictionary[11] the Latin stem of confabulation is a confabulari: (con), together, plus (fabulari) to talk or chat. Thus the root concerns talking together or familiar talk. There is no reference to falsifying or "making up" statements, which is one definition of fabrication,[12] a word used in the definition above. In medical entries in the residents' charts, confabulation has been made to be synonymous (which it is not) with fabrication, thereby carrying the latter's evaluative meaning—the implication of intent.

In contrast, the metaphor used by Arnella Smith describes the residents' intermittent change in coherency as a change in *direction*, with no attached evaluation. In the following statement, CNA Arnella talks about "going from drive into reverse":

> You can be talking to any one of the residents, and they're talking where you can understand quite well what they are saying. Then all of a sudden the thought just leaves their mind and they're talking about something entirely different. I don't really let on to them what they have done. I just go on and let them … they just go on and talk about what they're talking about now. I just look at it as them going from drive into reverse. But, one thing, you never walk away from them.

It is important not to miss or *dismiss*, the subtleties of meaning in Arnella's words. Her language can be interpreted on two levels. First, it is an example of the staff's attempt to uphold resident agency and provide emotional support. On another level, her words may serve the purpose of shielding a staff member's full recognition of a resident's cognitive loss. The staff see the resident "moving on over," in their words, to the third unit, an ominous sign of what they call the resident's "taking a turn" meaning ultimate and quick demise. It is important to remember that neither of these possibilities is "the" interpretation, nor are they mutually exclusive. Members of the staff appear to hold both in a delicate balance, which involves the tension of holding on and letting go.

What is the significance, beyond being an interesting artifact of local culture, of alternative language such as "keeping busy" instead of "wandering," "levels" instead of "stages," or "turning" instead of "going down"? The answer is twofold. First, there is the preservation of a measure of self-determination and control for the person with Alzheimer's disease. Second, there is a normalizing of the setting for the CNAs themselves that helps them to construct a "world of their own." The difference between saying an "Alzheimer's patient" (or worse, victim) and a "person with Alzheimer's disease" connotes a dramatic difference in helping maintain and acknowledge surviving facets of self.

Alternatives to Stage Theory

Representing the medical model of dementia, "Stage Theory"[13] is a major explanatory and descriptive framework which argues that there are discrete and discernable "stages" in Alzheimer's disease through which people pass before dying. The model is a theory that posits uni-linear progression of pathology in brain tissue[14] with no new learning taking place at each successive "stage" of the disease. Criticism of the theory has focused on its exclusion of the social and its hidden effort to create order, predictability, and control.

RN Elaine Pressley explains the use of stages in relation to the history of the structural set-up of the Pavilion:

> At first it was used to try to group people, but after a while everything that the residents did. How we all perceived them. We have had some where there were three stages and one where there were five stages depending on the things we were using. Somebody might fit into a group with their ADL[15] skills but then their mental and memory was in a different group. Take Elsie Kidd, for example. When she came in she could help take care of herself but when they did her memory evaluation it was three (low). So her skills with ADLs and helping herself didn't go with her memory.

RN Pressley reveals several things in this passage: an orientation to the individuality of residents in the start-up and running of the Pavilion; the reliance on, and primacy of empirical, indigenous knowledge; and, a use of the intuitive to organize social and medical aspects. Elaine Pressley also raises the issue of residents having multiple levels of functioning, all at the same time, that do not lend themselves to classification into categories.

All members of the staff in the Alzheimer's Pavilion at Starrmount have some degree of acquaintance with stage theory. Some speak of it as "standing for" a series of declines in the resident, necessitating their "ending up" on the non-ambulatory third unit in the Alzheimer's Pavilion. Others speak of the debate over the number and definition of stages. The staff's response to the theory contains seeds of ambiguity, complexity, skepticism, questions, and degrees of reframing based on their experiential knowledge. Members of the staff have their own constructs and signposts for evaluating and sensing a resident's need, as one puts it, "to move on" to the third unit. That need can occur when residents stop talking, are unable to eat, and, most significantly, become consistently incontinent. These changes in a resident's behavior are markers that also carry strong emotional valences, with respect to the probability that a resident will have to be "moved on." Focus is placed on the third unit, not because the care is deficient, quite the contrary, but because of what it symbolizes to the staff; they lose the emotional connection they had with that resident. A sense of finality sets in. Even though the spatial distance to the third unit is short, the changed self of the resident is now just out of reach. As Justine puts it when speaking about a favorite resident just transferred to the third unit, "She just isn't our Marge anymore." In addition, there is the changed identity of the staff from involved caregivers to bystanders.

Marita Martin's "scale of one to ten" is a personal schema that is relevant for her. She tells me, "That's just the way I categorize them. I would use this in evaluating the residents on a day-to-day basis." Her scale takes into account physical changes such as incontinence, eating, and sleeping habits. The scale also includes subtle behavioral changes, such as when a resident starts the process of "putting on and taking off shoes" during the day. Implicit in Marita's scale is an allowance for the potential effects of the social environment on the process of dementia. For example, Marita remarked to me that she is still uncertain about why and when the "whole shoe thing," started happening. Marita does not attribute the cause to the disease immediately, but gives thoughtful consideration and study to the expressions of the residents over time.

The "scale of one to ten" can be interpreted as a substitute for stage theory as a classification tool, but with significant differences: it is centered on the resident and situated within the context of the Pavilion; it is grounded in, and sensitive to, changes arising from the empirical world and is therefore more individualized; and, it is less rigid and shows more gradations than stage theory.

Another example of naming and reframing that conveys the sense of struggle associated with classifying people is the way CNA Carma thinks about stages. In the following statement, the "I," the acting self of the resident, speaks rather than the resident being cast as symptomatic object:

> Okay, the first level is the "I know everything," I'll call it. The second stage is … "I'm sorry." The first stage is "Okay, I know what kind of dress I want to wear. I know how to comb my hair, how to brush my teeth. I know how to take care of my own self." They're more self-dependent. That's the first level to me. The second level would be where they're not as talkative. They

> tend to depend more on the caregiver. The third level is when they're totally dependent on the caregiver.

In this example, Carma Lee places the person with Alzheimer's in the narrator's position. The resident speaks through a reflexive self that understands a question and defends the self as actor. In Carma's construction, the resident assumes a sense of identity, albeit briefly, at the locus of control: the true actor, still not completely "acted upon." Interestingly, she refers to the resident in the "first stage" as "self-dependent" rather than independent. Thus, the focus remains on the primacy of the singular identity of the resident; Carma reveals more about her own version of stage theory in her description of Ella Mason, an 82-year-old widow of independent spirit:

> Ella, for example. She's at the point where she can't really do anything for herself, but at the same time she doesn't want you to do it. When she first came here she was a little better. She could do more for herself, but now it's *almost* (my emphasis) second level because every day she gets so confused. If you assist her, she can do her socks. Brushing her teeth or hygiene, she can't do any more.

In the last part of Carma's remarks, there is almost the implication that, before the second stage, there is a chance to "get better," but once the resident reaches the second stage, it's all downhill. Carma begs the question of how one moves through discrete stages when she speaks of "almost" second stage and "going into" the third stage. Her wording suggests that the residents remain on the cusp of stages, or in the transitional areas, thereby confirming CNA Carma's reluctance to use a set of discrete stages and her ambivalence about classification lest it unfairly label the person. Carma Lee points out subtle distinctions in Ella Mason's dilemma of not being able to do certain things for herself but very hesitant to relinquish her "self-dependence" just as Carma may be hesitant to acknowledge "her" resident's inevitable decline.

Justine's response to stage theory also addresses the difficulty in defining discrete stages. She attests to remarkable individual variation among residents. Outward manifestations of change and deterioration may mask other enduring capacities, which are perceived by the CNAs who care for them on a daily basis. Justine makes the following observation:

> When we get a resident, they come in, they're walkin', they're talkin', they're feeding themselves. Basically a normal day. After three to six months, something changes. They may stop feeding themselves. I've seen them stop talking. Stop walking altogether. But yet they can listen to me when I say a thing to them, and it's like they know what I'm saying. They understand me. Then, they then have to move to the third unit.

Demonstrating her ability to make distinctions, Justine affirms her own expertise, her abilities to communicate where others may fail. Her reframing suggests variability, the ambiguity of stages, and the persistence of self-consciousness in a person who can understand what she is saying. She separates the resident's loss of ability to perform instrumental tasks from what she perceives in the social or interactive sense—the resident's capacity to listen and to understand her. There is a subtle, yet profound, difference between person as focal point and symptoms as focal point.

Justine designates a temporal aspect, three to six months as a benchmark when "something changes" in the residents, suggesting that she notices precipitous rather than incremental change during this interval. When in the middle of her comments, she mentions that they can still "understand her," there is almost an implicit question about the real significance of the other changes relative to their ability to understand her. She alludes to the following question: By what criteria do we place people in stages, especially when they may be functioning on different instrumental, cognitive, social, and physiological levels at the same time? Justine concludes with more explicit questions about the clarity of discrete stages:

> I don't know. A lot of ours that have been down here, maybe two or three years before. We try to say well, maybe something's just making them sick, maybe a urinary tract infection or a cold or something. We try to go along these lines first before we say that this is a part of the disease, "she's just got to move on."

Justine's narrative resembles a story depicting a journey, especially her use of lines "it's just time for her to leave" and "she's just got to move on." The reframing that is evident in her comments is akin to "leave-taking" from the family—an interpretation that is embedded in a relational context of collective membership. The emotional investment in the residents, and the resulting effects on the staff when they cannot "hold on" to the residents are hinted at in Justine's narrative.

The CNAs do not always agree with the decision to move a resident to the third unit, and they make this known. They want to preserve, even rehabilitate the resident, using the sociocultural context of the Pavilion to help the resident "come back." CNA Chevelle talks about what she calls "changes" in the residents:

> It's like at first they can go to the bathroom, they can do almost everything normal. Then you notice later on they've changed. They might start sleeping in the bed late something like they never normally do. Stuff like their movement started changing. Like they'll start picking at some part of the clothing, stuff like that. You could just see the change. They just take a whole different change. Then they start urinating on themselves. Stop eating. It just seems like they're going to another level. Sometimes they go back, though. Like Jane reminds me of that. Once she had stopped eating altogether. Then, before you know it, she's right back eating again. Like

> there was nothing ever wrong before. So maybe she forgot how to eat. Now, I've seen them do that too. They've come back. But most of the time it gets regressive. Usually a lot of them end up over there (arching her neck toward the Third Unit doors, while not turning to face them). That's their last level.

For Chevelle, there is the possibility of a resident "coming back to *themselves*" or recovering what seemed to be a lost capacity. CNAs may not see or may not *want* to see the inevitability of the disease and therefore entertain the thought that they can "bring um back" if given a chance. For Chevelle, the reframing in her narrative takes the form of a mixture of "regression" and the intermittent return of former abilities. She does not have a deterministic view of the disease and allows for other possibilities. Whether that is medically reconcilable, Chevelle's view may allow for a different engagement with the resident, having the effect of what staff prioritize as "maintaining a person's emotional well-being."

The staff view levels as contextually situated. That is, they see levels as connected with the designation and set-up of their own Pavilion grounded in the idiosyncrasies of each person. Levels I and II evolved, in part, according to the residents' "preferences," as Unit Manager Pressley explains. Thus, stages do not have the same meanings for the staff as they do in the medical model. Most members of the staff would appear to agree with the position that there is much inconsistency in what signifies moving from one stage to another.

In a halting manner, Unit Manager Elaine Pressley expresses her quandary about the use of stage theory:

> I wonder if you would sometimes … if they would … would you be willing—I don't know what I want to say—expect sometimes—a particular stage but they might be higher functioning. Would you expect less of them or "down" them? Do you know what I mean?

Two important things are apparent regarding the language of openings and the naming and reframing process. First, they preserve a measure of self-control and agency for the residents. Second, they put the locus of control and degrees of power on the Pavilion in the hands of the staff based upon their knowledge.

To create meaning and to gain knowledge in an amorphous scene with residents who are complex is not an easy task. Yet, there is the impetus among the staff to possess knowledge of the human beings before them. Among other reasons, this impetus may emanate from their desire to make their work more meaningful to *themselves*. Bed and body work can become routine and unchallenging over time, precisely what the CNAs reject. Caring for the residents is an involved process that takes initiative and mental energy to gather knowledge, store it, build on it, and apply it, the same *process* that highly educated medical practitioners do in the practice of their professions.[16]

Notes

1 James Scott, *Seeing Like a State: How Certain Schemes to Improve the Human Condition Have Failed* (New Haven, CT: Yale University Press, 1998: 6).

2 Marcel Detienne and Claude Vernant, *Cunning Intelligence in Greek Culture and Society*, trans. Janet Lloyd (Atlantic Highlands, NJ: Humanities Press, 1978), originally published in French as *Les ruses d'intelligence:La metis des grecs* (Paris: Flammarion, 1974) provide one of the most thorough and illuminating tomes on the history and practice of *Metis*. They seek to impress upon us that "Such intelligence involves several kinds of levels one of which is … the cunning stratagems of war, frauds, deceits, resourcefulness of every kind" (Detienne and Vernant 1978: 11); it implies a complex but very coherent body of mental attitudes and intellectual behavior. I thank Robert Emerson for introducing me to James Scott's work, *Seeing Like a State*, and the concept of *Metis*, which subsequently led me to the original work on *Metis* by Detienne and Vernant.

3 James C. Scott, *Seeing Like a State: How Certain Schemes to Improve the Human Condition Have Failed* (New Haven, CT: Yale University Press, 1998: 313–315).

4 According to Michael Polanyi, *Knowing and Being* (Chicago, IL: University of Chicago Press, 1969: 159),

> Tacit knowing involves arriving at knowledge through internal reflection. It is something we cannot verify or explain or account for; it just is. The knowledge is tacit, a whole, and cannot be broken into aspects or parts.

This grasping of wholes is illustrated by Marita Martin's description of what she senses as an aura.

5 Michael Polanyi, *The Tacit Dimension* (Gloucester, MA: Peter Smith Publishers, 1967: 182). For recent research, see Pia Kontos and Gary Naglie, "Tacit Knowledge of Caring and Embodied Selfhood," *Sociology of Health and Illness* 31 (2009): 688–704.

6 Audre Lorde, *Sister Outsider: Essays and Speeches* (Freedom, CA: The Crossing Press, 1984).

7 James C. Scott, *Seeing Like a State: How Certain Schemes to Improve the Human Condition Have Failed* (New Haven, CT: Yale University Press, 1998: 316).

8 Medical sociologist Irving Zola, "Bringing Our Bodies and Ourselves Back in: Reflections on a Past, Present, and Future Medical Sociology," *Journal of Health and Social Behavior* 3 (1991): 14 comments on the shift of control when he talks about the language of disability:

> They (prepositions) imply both a relationship to and a separation from. Thus, in describing an individual's relationship to an assistive device such as a wheelchair, the difference between "being confined to" a wheelchair and "using" a wheelchair is a difference not only in terminology but in control.

See also Irving Zola, "The Naming Question: Reflections on the Language of Disability," in *Report of the American Association for the Advancement of Science Workshop on the Demography of Scientists and Engineers with Disabilities* (Washington, DC: American Association for the Advancement of Science, 1992). Marita Martin was not ready to "lock in" a name for Abe Steck's condition with its potential negative repercussions for Abe's self-identity.

9 Karen A. Lyman, "Bringing the Social Back In: A Critique of the Biomedicalization of Dementia," *The Gerontologist* 5 (1989): 597–605.

10 *Dorland's Illustrated Medical Dictionary* (2011: 368).

11 Oxford English Dictionary (OED) (2011: 509).
12 Ibid.
13 For a discussion of medicine's seven-stage theory of Alzheimer's disease, see Barry Reisberg et al., "The BEHAVE-AD Assessment System, a Perspective, a Commentary on New Findings, and a Historical Review," *Dementia and Geriatric Cognitive Disorders* 38 (2014): 1–2. See also, the definition and use of a three-stage theory model, *Alzheimer's Association*, 2017.
14 Tom Kitwood, "The Dialectics of Dementia: With Particular Reference to Alzheimer's Disease," *Ageing and Society* 10 (1990): 177–196.
15 The Activities of Daily Living (ADLs) assessment instrument was originally developed by Duke University to determine the functional conditions of elders compared to others in their cohort. According to Michelle Mlinac and Michelle Feng, "Assessment of Activities of Daily Living, Self Care, and Independence," *Activities of Clinical Neuropsychology* 31 (2016): 506, ADLs are "basic actions that involve caring for one's body and self, including personal care, mobility and eating."
16 On an important methodological note, psychoanalyst Heinz Kohut coined the terms "experience-near" and "experience-distant" concepts in his work, which were appropriated by anthropologist Clifford Geertz for use in anthropological interpretation: Geertz, Clifford, *Local Knowledge: Further Essays in Interpretive Anthropology* (New York: Basic Books, 1983). Geertz (pg. 57) explains,

> An experience-near concept is, roughly, one that someone … an informant—might himself naturally and effortlessly use to define what he or his fellows see, feel, think, imagine … and which he would readily understand when similarly applied by others …

"Getting into the resident's world" is an experience-near conceptual phrase, as are "going into the zone" and "taking a turn," among others that the CNAs and Marita Martin use to make sense of their world. An experience-distant concept, according to Geertz, is

> one that specialists of one sort or another … employ to forward their scientific, practical aims … "Social stratification" and perhaps for most peoples in the world even "religion" (and certainly "religious system") are experience-distant.

These critical distinctions have been central to my analysis in remaining faithful to respondents' own terms by which they describe their world while moving beyond description alone to interpretation.

CONCLUSION

This book provides a revealing glimpse into the social construction of a culture of care. In the book's opening scene, CNA Justine King confronts a substitute CMT (Certified Medical Technician) who is accusing resident Marge Jacobs of spitting on her. Justine comes with a question, "Just what happened here?" The substitute aide answers, "she spit on me." Justine responds, "Well I don't know if she did or not but we don't talk to our residents the way you just did. No sir-ee. We, ah, do things just a LIT...tle differently down here." "When you come on our floor, you got to respect us, you got to respect our residents." Rather than assigning "blame," Justine moves immediately toward a strategy and philosophy of care work.

Care, whether viewed as acts of civility, acts of compassion and skill, or acts of close personal interaction, is the fundamental process by which society perpetuates and recreates itself. Care work in the United States and other affluent nations, is subject to an interesting irony. On the one hand, this work is highly valued by the individuals who benefit, and it receives generic cultural support (i.e. positive "lip service" that expresses regard for care work); yet, at the same time, this work is devalued in that paid care workers garner little in the way of public recognition or compensation. Jobs such as nursing assistant, home health aide, and child daycare worker are increasingly vital to the quality of life for millions of older persons and young children, making possible successful social and economic arrangements within many American families. Despite social need and the undeniable benefit of these occupations, workers in such positions face low pay and a notable lack of social status. These contradictions have received modest attention in public policy discussion, with very limited inclusion of how the circumstances of care work are revealed in the perspectives of paid care workers themselves.

The Helen Wise Pavilion at Starrmount Geriatric might appear to be primarily a place of undefined activity and movement, with so-called "meaningful" life in absentia. Yet, an engaging, complex world of care, meaning and struggle lies just below all appearances. The Pavilion is an amalgam of energies. There are those generated by the residents living out the whole of their lives in this place, under this care, day and night. There is also energy of a distinctive, absorbing kind generated by staff as they respond to two formative tasks: performing manifold duties for the residents and keeping alive the vision and practice of their care.

Autonomy

Certified Nursing Assistants, when given levels of autonomy in their work in an institution, forge a "different" model of care work.[1] Degrees of Freedom, making lives meaningful, and the ongoing reassurance of the residents' emotional well-being that the CNAs talk about are multifaceted in expression. Out of the fundamental philosophy of the Alzheimer's Pavilion, set forth by a collaboration of nursing and social services, Marita Martin and her team of CNAs have given teeth and dimension to the original over time.

CNAs and LPN Marita Martin engage in various processes which produce meaningfully personal care by CNAs in the kind of nursing home situation that is synonymous with impersonal, non-caring treatment. They have constructed their own ethic, practice, and body of knowledge in their own terms. Those terms consist, importantly, of a language of care, what they call "our own little language," a skill that they use to create diverse channels of communication which they call, "getting into the resident's world." Staff work in multiple realities every day and must bridge those disparate realities between and among staff and residents. The Pavilion is a fluid milieu where residents are free to express their individuality with minimal pressure to conform and have the opportunity to make choices and express preferences. In this world, caregiving is rooted in, and rises out of two things: the relationship between staff and residents and, vitally important, the relationship among the CNAs themselves.

CNAs and Marita Martin have a respect and concern for each other. There is collective sentiment, equality and loyalty on a practical as well as a deeply intuitive level among the staff, a solidarity from Durkheim's perspective where moral decision-making arises from teamwork relationships. From Mead's perspective, the selves of care workers and residents and the society in this Pavilion are "twin born" and mutually dependent. Care is ontologically relational and can only be understood within these connections.

Frontline staff construct the meaning of their work and identities through forms of resistance manifested through their development, ownership and execution of a privileged knowledge of the residents, which serves as an alternative script to the hegemonic medical model of health care; through their expression of working-class agency and efforts to create a world for themselves and residents as a reaction to the bureaucratized structure of which they are a part; and to the macro urban environment with its racism, sexism, inequality, and through their "staying power" on the Pavilion where positive meaning associated with their labor is both tough and fragile. They desire to create a world that is the antithesis of the world in which they live on the outside.

The context in which staff operate is both a refuge and a site of struggle. The staff seek to create a haven, a "self place" for themselves and the residents. Theirs is an active, not passive one, however, where the staff are advocates trying to give voice to residents and themselves. I argue that advocacy for the residents has a sense of vicarious satisfaction: a channel for their own grievances associated with it. Fisher[2] talks of caring as being the "work of maintaining and repairing ourselves and the world." In a vital sense, the CNAs and Marita Martin are attempting to repair themselves and the residents as the latter affirms:

> There is a hesitation for all of us to go out that door. It's like an island, a refuge. Our wants and needs, I think are met here with the Alzheimer's residents. I haven't had very good relationships with people and I have always clung to my job and always given 200%. That gratifies me. The caring part is so euphoric to me that sometimes I drive myself crazy over it because I like feeling like that. I think the girls have that like I do because they're happy when they know that somebody's well-cared for or somebody comes by and says, "She looks great today," and it's a euphoria for them. That's my name on that resident.

While the "Island Feeling" serves constructive, creative functions for residents and staff, it also expresses a counter side, a "site of struggle." The warp and woof of demanding care work, the tension staff feel toward the administration and its representatives, rules and regulations, the ever-present bureaucratic routinization and temporal regularity, blatant racism from a resident, as well as intrusions on their autonomy from families and the medical enterprise, are daily strains. CNAs harbor frustration over the lack of official recognition (in the charts and by the public) of the range and level of their knowledge, which functions as the fulcrum on which the Pavilion operates. Carma Lee speaks for the CNAs:

> My biggest problem is with administration. They can show all the in-service they want. They can even pay all the money they want. But, if they're not there to see what's going on ... They're not doing their part. Your self-esteem goes back down ... Motivation is affected. They don't understand what you go through. It is very demanding sometimes. No one seems to care.

It is not just observing their labor that the CNAs consistently speak of, but also the administration's bearing witness to their care.

Confluence of Factors

One can be given autonomy and do nothing with it. How might we come to understand the confluence of factors that contributed to the construction of the Starrmount CNAs' care world?

From the beginning, Starrmount Alzheimer's Pavilion was imbued with a special status because it was the first of its kind in the area and thought of as the best. In addition to the relative autonomy that the CNAs experienced, the CNAs also felt that the special status of the Pavilion on the micro-level was reinforced, on the macrostructural level, by the public perception of Alzheimer's disease as the "worst of all diseases," demanding extraordinary attention. In addition, Marita Martin's experience as a CNA, her psychiatric background, her leadership of the Pavilion and her relationship with the RN manager were critical to the positive development of the program.

These factors are necessary, but not sufficient, to explain the world of care they constructed. The CNAs' impetus to create an ideal world and their team relationship were needed. Staff took the initiative and were mindful. They spoke of other floors as having such a fast pace. In the Pavilion, it was more subtle. One CNA remarked that "The time kind of stands still. On the other floors, we're constantly taking vitals. On the Alzheimer's Pavilion, no one really calls for you, so it was a whole new ballgame for me."

Staff realized that the momentum of the individual is to hold onto fragments of self and identity throughout the life course. This drive may assume heightened intensity with the onslaught of multiple physical and social compromises of old age. Behavior that is viewed as disruptive may, in fact, be a way of claiming a measure of agency and control.

Implications

Along with more staff autonomy, a language of alternative practices to the medical model can be transformative of institutional care and care work in general. This detailed language and practice of care, though often unrecognized, can substitute for the bureaucratic language that doesn't recognize patients' complexity.

As part of revolutionary change, new language can be introduced into the analysis of workplace social relations in care work and considered in depth in future research. Concepts could include creativity, worker initiative and pride, socially constructed knowledge, emotional wellbeing, dignity, insider/local knowledge, team support/ensemble, administrative exploitation, worker resistance, autonomy, ethic of care and advocacy. Structural factors such as ratio of staff to residents, staff training programs, and staff turnover affect the caliber of caregiving; however, they represent the more obvious factors. This research suggests a deeper level that examines the underlying assumptions of care. We tend to dichotomize planning and meaning just as we tend to compartmentalize provision of care, the relationship in which it is forged, and the ethic and philosophy that informs it. We must decompartmentalize these issues and illuminate their mutual influence on one another in settings where mutuality is most crucial to understand.

Concentrating less on how to manage the patient's behavior, and more on what premise informs the work makes sense because assumptions are manifested in the details, in the descriptive language of care. Diamond[3] describes what Starrmount staff have demonstrated in their "own little language" and body of knowledge and skills. He states:

> Mother's wit and its narrative based in caretaking is not a priority list of changes that need to be made but the illumination of a base of knowledge from which they can be made. It is a constant and widespread set of practices. It is more than an attitude, more than a set of invisible skills, and more than coordinating the internal and external forces. Since it is all of these, it can be a base for a revolutionary set of practices.

Historically, we have neglected what low-level workers, often women of color, can provide, because we have succumbed to the stereotype of these workers as passive and lacking in agency, not relevant to research agendas.[4] As we study care workers, we can come to understand autonomy on a continuum and the kind of resistance that can express itself as positive forms of agency on the part of those least expected to have it. This study challenges traditional ideas in the working-class literature that more supervision provides the best quality of work for CNAs. The CNAs and LPN charge nurse at Starrmount are cultivating an identity as women of color who are engaged in service work that is socially responsible work. Frontline workers (mostly women) are the most crucial providers, after informal caregivers, in the long-term care system. In the case of the Starrmount CNAs, staff express wanting to be in their job of providing mindful care. At the same time they want to participate in a larger world where they and their work are respected and fairly valued.

Notes

1 In response to Nancy Foner's query, *The Caregiving Dilemma: Work in an American Nursing Home* (Berkeley, CA: University of California Press, 1995).
2 Berenice Fisher, "Alice in the Human Services: A Feminist Analysis of Women in the Caring Professions," in Emily Abel and Margaret Nelson (eds), *Circles of Care: Work and Identity in Women's Lives* (Albany, NY: State University of New York, 1990: 111).
3 Timothy Diamond, *Making Gray Gold: Narratives of Nursing Home Care* (Chicago, IL and London: University of Chicago Press, 1992: 242).
4 Sharon Harley, "Speaking Up: The Politics of Black Women's Labor History," in Elizabeth Higginbotham and Mary Romero (eds), *Women and Work: Exploring Race, Ethnicity, and Class* (Thousand Oaks, CA: Sage Publications, 1997: 28–52). Harley speaks about a "hidden history of black working class agency." She argues there is so little research on this because "Their low status jobs and assumption of low working class consciousness, made poor women of color unworthy of research."

BIBLIOGRAPHY

Abel, Emily, and Margaret Nelson. 1990. "Circles of Care: An Introductory Essay." In Emily Abel and Margaret Nelson (eds), *Circles of Care: Work and Identity in Women's Lives*. Albany, NY: State University of New York Press, 1990: 4–34.

Addis, Donna, and Lynette J. Tippett. 2004. "Memory of Myself: Autobiographical Memory and Identity in Alzheimer's Disease." *Memory* 12: 56–74.

Alzheimer's Disease Facts and Figures Report. 2017.

American Geriatrics Core Writing Group. 2010. S251.

Banaszak-Holl, Jane, and Marilyn A. Hines. 1996. "Factors Associated with Nursing Home Staff Turnover." *Gerontologist* 36: 512–517.

Barbour, Allen. 1995. *Caring for Patients: A Critique of the Medical Model*. Palo Alto, CA: Stanford University Press.

Barnes, Marian. 2012. *Care in Everyday Life: An Ethics of Care in Practice*. Bristol: The Policy Press.

Barnes, Marian, and Tula Brannelly (eds). 2015. *Ethics of Care: Critical Advances in International Perspective*. Bristol: The Policy Press.

Beard, Renée. 2004. "In Their Voices: Identity Preservation and Experiences of Alzheimer's Disease." *Journal of Aging Studies* 18: 415–428.

Benner, Patricia, and Suzanne Gordon. 1996. "Caring Practice." In Suzanne Gordon, Patricia Benner and Nel Noddings (eds), *Caregiving: Readings in Knowledge, Practice, Ethics, and Politics*. Philadelphia, PA: University of Pennsylvania Press: 40–53.

Bentham, Jeremy. 1995. *The Panopticon Writings*. Edited by Miran Bozovic. London: Verso: 29.

Berdes, Celia, and John M. Eckert. 2001. "Race Relations and Caregiving Relationships: A Qualitative Perspective from Residents and Aides in Three Nursing Homes." *Research on Aging* 23: 109–126.

———. 2007. "The Language of Caring: Nurse's Aides' Use of Family Metaphors Conveys Affective Care." *Gerontologist* 47: 340–349.

Berger, Peter, and Thomas Luckmann. 1967. *The Social Construction of Reality: A Treatise in the Sociology of Knowledge*. New York: Anchor Press: 21, 23, 25.

Blum, Nancy. 1994. "Deceptive Practices in Managing a Family Member with Alzheimer's Disease." *Symbolic Interaction* 17: 21–36.

Blumer, Herbert. 1936. "Social Attitudes and Nonsymbolic Interaction." *Journal of Educational Sociology* 9: 517.

———. 1986. *Symbolic Interaction: Perspective and Method*. Oakland, CA: University of California Press.

Bogdan, Robert, and Steven Carter. 1992. "The Social Construction of Humanness: Relationships with Severely Disabled People." *Interpreting Disability: A Qualitative Reader* 7: 275–294.

Bogdan, Robert, and Steven Taylor. 1974. "Let Them Eat Programs: Attendants' Perspectives and Programming in Wards in State Schools." *Journal of Health and Social Behavior* 15: 142–150.

———. 1987. "Toward a Sociology of Acceptance: The Other Side of the Study of Deviance." *Social Policy* 18: 3

Bubeck, Diemut. 1995. *Care, Gender and Justice*. Oxford: Clarendon Press: 129.

Cancian, Francesca M. 2000. "Paid Emotional Care." In Madonna Harrington Meyer (ed), *Care Work: Gender, Labor, and the Welfare State*. New York: Routledge: 136–148.

Castle, Nicholas G., and John Engberg. 2006. "Organizational Characteristics Associated with Staff Turnover in Nursing Homes." *Gerontologist* 46: 62–73.

Caudell, Lisa, and Linda Clare. 2010. "The Impact of Dementia on Self and Identity." *Clinical Psychology Review* 20: 113–126.

Chambliss, Daniel. 1996. *Beyond Caring: Hospitals, Nurses and the Social Organization of Ethics*. Chicago, IL: University of Chicago Press: 40.

Cohen-Mansfield, Jiska, Aleksandra Parpura-Gill, and Hava Golander. 2006. "Salience of Self-Identity Roles in Persons with Dementia: Difference in Perceptions among Elderly Persons, Family Members, and Caregivers." *Social Science and Medicine* 62: 745–757.

Collins, Patricia Hill. 1986. "Learning from the Outsider Within: The Sociological Significance of Black Feminist Thought." *Social Problems* 33: S25.

Davis, Daniel. 2004. "Dementia: Sociological and Philosophical Constructions." *Social Science and Medicine* 58: 369–378.

Detienne, Marcel, and Claude Vernant. 1978. *Cunning Intelligence in Greek Culture and Society*. Translated by Janet Lloyd. Atlantic Highlands, NJ: Humanities Press, 1978. Originally published in French as *Les ruses d'intelligence: La metis des grecs*. Paris: Flammarion, 1974.

DeVault, Marjorie L. 1994. *Feeding the Family: The Social Organization of Caring as Gendered Work*. Chicago, IL: University of Chicago Press.

Diamond, Timothy. 1992. *Making Gray Gold: Narratives of Nursing Home Care*. Chicago, IL and London: University of Chicago Press.

Dodson, Lisa, and Rebekah Zincavage. 2007. "It's Like a Family: Caring Labor, Exploitation, and Race in Nursing Homes." *Gender and Society* 21: 905–928.

Dorland's Illustrated Medical Dictionary. 2011, pg. 368.

Duffy, Mignon, Amy Armenia, and Clare Stacey (eds). 2015. *Caring on the Clock: The Complexities and Contradictions of Paid Care Work*. New Brunswick, NJ: Rutgers University Press.

Durkheim, Emile. 2008 [1912]. *Elementary Forms of Religious Life*. Edited by Mark S. Cladis and translated from the French by Carol Cosman. New York: Oxford University Press.

Emerson, Robert, and Sheldon Messinger. 1977. "The Micro-Politics of Trouble." *Social Problems* 25: 121–134.

Emerson, Robert, Rachel Fretz, and Linda Shaw. 2011. *Writing Ethnographic Fieldnotes*. Chicago, IL: University of Chicago Press.

England, Paula. 2005. "Emerging Theories of Care Work." *Annual Review of Sociology* 31: 381–399.

England, Paula, Michelle Budig, and Nancy Folbre. 2002. "Wages of Virtue: The Relative Pay of Care Work." *Social Problems* 49: 455–473.

Estes, Carroll, and Elizabeth Binney. 1989. "The Biomedicalization of Aging: Dangers and Dilemmas." *Gerontologist* 29: 587–596.

Fazio, Sam, and David B. Mitchell. 2009. "Persistence of Self in Individuals with Alzheimer's Disease." *Dementia* 8: 39–59.

Fisher, Berenice. 1990. "Alice in the Human Services: A Feminist Analysis of Women in the Caring Professions." In Emily Abel and Margaret Nelson (eds), *Circles of Care: Work and Identity in Women's Lives.* Albany, NY: State University of New York Press: 111.

Folbre, Nancy. 2001. *The Invisible Heart: Economics and Family Values.* New York: New Press.

Foner, Nancy. 1995. *The Caregiving Dilemma: Work in an American Nursing Home.* Berkeley, CA: University of California Press.

Foucault, Michel. 1973. *The Birth of the Clinic: An Archeology of Medical Perception.* New York: Vintage.

———. 1980. *Power/Knowledge.* New York: Pantheon Books: 81.

Geertz, Clifford. 1983. *Local Knowledge: Further Essays in Interpretive Anthropology.* New York: Basic Books.

———. 2017. *The Interpretation of Cultures.* New York: Basic Books.

Goffman, Erving. 1961. *Asylums.* New York: Anchor.

———. 1969. "The Insanity of Place." *Psychiatry: Journal for the Study of Interpersonal Processes* XXXII: 362, 366.

Gordon, Suzanne, Patricia Benner, and Nel Noddings (eds) 1996. *Caregiving: Readings in Knowledge, Practice, Ethics, and Politics.* Philadelphia, PA: University of Pennsylvania Press.

Graham, Hilary. 1983. "Caring: A Labor of Love." In Janet Finch and Dulcie Groves (eds), *A Labor of Love: Women, Work and Caring.* London: Routledge & Kegan Paul: 13–30.

Gubrium, Jaber F. 1975. *Living and Dying at Murray Manor.* New York: St. Martin's Press.

———. 1986. *Oldtimers and Alzheimers: The Descriptive Organization of Senility.* Greenwich, CT: JAI Press.

———. 1986. "The Social Preservation of Mind: The Alzheimer's Disease Experience." *Symbolic Interaction* 9: 37–51.

Gubrium, Jaber F., and David Buckholdt. 1982. *Fictive Family: Everyday Usage, Analytic, and Human Service Considerations.* Hoboken, NJ: Wiley-Blackwell: 878–885.

Gubrium, Jaber F., and James Holstein. 1990. *What is Family?* Houston, TX: Mayfield Publishing: ix–x.

Gubrium, Jaber F., and Margaretha Järvinen (eds). 2014. *Turning Troubles into Problems: Clientization in Human Services.* London: Routledge.

Gubrium, Jaber F., and Robert Lynott. 1987. "Measurement and the Interpretation of Burden in the Alzheimer's Disease Experience." *Journal of Aging Studies* 1: 265–285.

Gubrium, Jaber F., Tone Alm Andreassen, and Per Koren (eds). 2016. *Reimagining the Human Service Relationship.* New York: Columbia University Press.

Habermas, Jürgen. 1991. *Moral Consciousness and Communicative Action.* Cambridge, MA: MIT Press: 24.

Harley, Sharon. 1997. "Speaking Up: The Politics of Black Women's Labor History." In Elizabeth Higginbotham and Mary Romero (eds), *Women and Work: Exploring Race, Ethnicity, and Class.* Thousand Oaks, CA: Sage Publications: 28–51.

Harrington Meyer, Madonna (ed.) 2000. *Care Work: Gender, Class, and the Welfare State.* New York: Routledge.

Hayes, Jeanne, Craig Boylstein, and Mary K. Zimmerman. 2009. "Living and Loving with Dementia: Negotiating Spousal and Caregiver Identity Through Narrative." *Journal of Aging Studies* 23: 48–59.

Hayes, Jeanne, Mary K. Zimmerman, and Craig Boylstein. 2010. "Responding to Symptoms of Alzheimer's Disease: Husbands, Wives, and the Gendered Dynamics of Recognition and Disclosure." *Qualitative Health Research* 20: 1101–1115.

Held, Virginia. 2006. *The Ethics of Care: Personal, Political, and Global.* New York: Oxford University Press.

Henderson, Neil, and Maria Vesperi (eds). 1995. *The Culture of Long Term Care: Nursing Home Ethnography.* Westport, CT: Praeger.

Hochschild, Arlie. 1975. "The Sociology of Feeling and Emotion: Selected Possibilities." In Marcia Millman and Rosabeth Moss Cantor (eds), *In Another Voice: Feminist Perspectives on Social Life and Social Science.* Garden City, NY: Anchor/Doubleday Press: 280–307.

———. 1983. *The Managed Heart: Commercialization of Human Feeling.* Berkeley, CA: University of California Press.

———. 1989. *The Second Shift: Working Parents and the Revolution at Home.* New York: Viking Penguin.

Hodson, Randy. 2001. *Dignity at Work.* Cambridge: Cambridge University Press: 723.

Hodson, Randy, and Victor Roscigno. 1995. "Worker Resistance: An Underdeveloped Concept in the Sociology of Work." *Economic and Industrial Democracy* 16: 79–110.

Hughes, Everett. 1962. "Good People and Dirty Work." *Social Problems* 10: 3–11.

Illich, Ivan, Irving Zola, and John McKnight. 2000. *Disabling Professions.* London: Marian Boyers Publishers LTD.

Kayser-Jones, Jeanie. 1981. *Old, Alone and Neglected.* Berkeley, CA: University of California Press.

Kemp, Candace, Mary M. Ball, Molly Perkins, Carole Hollingsworth, and Michael J. Lepore. 2009. "'I Get Along With Most of Them': Direct Care Workers' Relationships with Residents' Families in Assisted Living." *Gerontologist* 49: 224–235.

Kittay, Eva Feder. 1999. *Love's Labor: Essays on Women, Equality, and Dependency.* New York: Routledge.

Kitwood, Tom. 1990. "The Dialectics of Dementia: With Particular Reference to Alzheimer's Disease." *Ageing and Society* 10: 177–196.

———. 1997. *Dementia Reconsidered: The Person Comes First.* Buckingham: Open University Press.

Kontos, Pia. 2004. "Ethnographic Reflections on Selfhood, Embodiment and Alzheimer's Disease." *Aging and Society* 24: 829–849.

Kontos, Pia, and Gary Naglie. 2009. "Tacit Knowledge of Caring and Embodied Selfhood." *Sociology of Health and Illness* 31: 688–704.

Lamont, Michelle, and Virag Molnar. 2002. "The Study of Boundaries in the Social Sciences." *Annual Review of Sociology* 28: 167–195.

Lofland, John, and Lyn Lofland. 1994. *Analyzing Social Settings.* Boston, MA: Cengage.

Lopez, Steven. 2006. "Emotional Labor and Organized Emotional Care: Conceptualizing Nursing Home Care Work." *Work and Occupations* 33: 133–160.

Lorber, Judith. 1995. "Night to his Day: The Social Construction of Gender." In *Paradoxes of Gender.* New Haven, CT: Yale University Press: 13–36.

Lorde, Audre. 1984. *Sister Outsider: Essays and Speeches.* Freedom, CA: The Crossing Press.

Lyman, Karen. 1988. "Infantilization of Elders: Day Care for Alzheimer's Disease Victims." In D. Wertz (ed), *Research in the Sociology of Health Care.* Greenwich, CT: JAI: 71–103.

———. 1989. "Bringing the Social Back In: A Critique of the Biomedicalization of Dementia." *Gerontologist* 29: 597–605.

Madden, Connie, Margaret Clayton, Heather E. Canary, Gail Towsley, Kristin Cloyes, and Dale Lund. 2017. "Rules of Performance in the Nursing Home: A Grounded Theory of Nurse–CNA Communication." *Geriatric Nursing* 38: 378–384.

Mead, George Herbert. 1934. *Mind, Self and Society: From the Standpoint of a Social Behaviorist.* Chicago, IL: University of Chicago Press.

Miller, Susan C., Edward Alan Miller, Hye-Young Jung, Samantha Sterns, Melissa Clark, and Vincent Mor. 2010. "Nursing Home Organizational Change: The 'Culture Change' Movement as Viewed by Long-Term Care Specialists." *Medical Care Research and Review* 67: 65S–81S.

Mishler, Elliot G. 1986. *Research Interviewing: Context and Narrative.* Cambridge, MA: Harvard University Press.

Mishler, Elliot G., Lorne R. Amarasingham, Samuel D. Osherson, Stuart T. Hauser, Nancy E. Waxler, and Ramsay Liem. 1981. *Social Contexts of Health and Illness, and Patient Care.* New York: Cambridge University Press.

Mlinac, Michelle, and Michelle Feng. 2016. "Assessment of Activities of Daily Living, Self Care, and Independence." *Activities of Clinical Neuropsychology* 31: 506.

Mol, Annemarie. 2008. *The Logic of Care: Health and the Problem of Patient Choice.* London: Routledge.

Nakano-Glen, Evelyn. 1985. "Racial Ethnic Women's Labor: The Intersection of Race, Gender and Class Oppression." *Review of Radical Political Economics* 17: 86–108.

———. 2000. "Creating a Caring Society." *Contemporary Sociology* 29: 84–94.

———. 2010. *Forced to Care: Coercion and Caregiving in America.* Cambridge, MA: Harvard University Press.

Occupational Outlook Handbook. 2011–2012. Bureau of Labor Statistics.

Oxford English Dictionary. 2011. pg. 509.

Parmelee, Patricia, Mary Laszio, and Jo Taylor. 2009. "Perceived Barriers to Effective Job Performance Among Nursing Assistants in Long-term Care." *Journal of the American Medical Directors Association* 10: 559–556.

Paules, Greta Foff. 1991. *Dishing It Out: Power and Resistance Among Waitresses in a New Jersey Restaurant.* Philadelphia, PA: Temple University Press.

Pekkarinen, Laura, Timo Sinervo, Marja-Leena Perala, and Marko Elovainio. 2004. "Work Stressors and the Quality of Life in Long-Term Care Units." *Gerontologist* 44: 633–643.

Pennington, Karen, Jill Scott, and Kathy Magilvy. 2003. "The Role of Certified Nursing Assistants in Nursing Homes." *Journal of Nursing Administration* 33: 578–584.

Polanyi, Michael. 1967. *The Tacit Dimension.* Gloucester, MA: Peter Smith Publishers: 182.

———. 1969. *Knowing and Being.* Chicago, IL: University of Chicago Press: 159.

Rahman, Anna N., and John F. Schnelle. 2008. "The Nursing Home Culture-Change Movement: Recent, Past, and Future Directions for Research." *Gerontologist* 48: 142–148.

Reach, Gerard. 2016. "Simplistic and Complex Thought in Medicine: The Rationale for a Person-Centered Care Model as a Medical Revolution." *Patient Preference and Adherence* 10: 449–457.

Reisberg, Barry. 1983. *Alzheimer's Disease.* New York: Free Press.

Reisberg, Barry, et al. 2014. "The BEHAVE-AD Assessment System, A Perspective, a Commentary on New Findings, and a Historical Review." *Dementia and Geriatric Cognitive Disorders* 38: 1–2.

Rodriquez, Jason. 2014. *Labors of Love: Nursing Homes and the Structures of Care Work.* New York: New York University Press.

———. 2011. "It's a Dignity Thing': Nursing Home Care Workers' Use of Emotions." *Sociological Forum* 26: 265–286.

Sabat, Steven. 2001. *The Experience of Alzheimer's Disease: Life Through a Tangled Veil.* Malden, MA: Blackwell Publishers.

Sabat, Steven, and Michelle Collins. 1999. "Intact Social, Cognitive Ability, and Selfhood: A Case Study of Alzheimer's Disease." *American Journal of Alzheimer's Disease* 14: 17.

Sabat, Steven, and Rom Harre. 1992. "The Construction and Deconstruction of Self in Alzheimer's Disease." *Aging and Society* 12: 269–287.

Savishinsky, Jay. 1991. *The Ends of Time: Life and Work in a Nursing Home.* New York: Bergin and Garvey.

Scheff, Thomas. 1999. *Being Mentally Ill: A Sociological Theory*. Piscataway, NJ: Aldine Transaction Publishers.

Schutz, Alfred. 1970. *The Phenomenology of the Social World.* Evanston, IL: Northwestern University Press.

Scott, James C. 1998. *Seeing Like a State: How Certain Schemes to Improve the Human Condition Have Failed.* New Haven, CT: Yale University Press: 6.

———. 1987. *Weapons of the Weak: Everyday Forms of Peasant Resistance.* New Haven, CT: Yale University Press: 292.

Shield, Renée. 1988. *Uneasy Endings: Daily Life in an American Nursing Home.* Ithaca, NY: Cornell University Press.

Simmel, Georg. 1955. *Conflict and The Web of Group Affiliation.* New York: The Free Press: 15–17.

Slote, Michael. 2007. *The Ethics of Care and Empathy.* London: Routledge.

Spradley, James. 1979. *The Ethnographic Interview.* Chicago, IL: Holt, Rinehart and Winston.

———. 1980. *Participant Observation.* Chicago, IL: Holt, Rinehart and Winston.

Stacey, Clare. 2005. "Finding Dignity in Dirty Work: The Constraints and Rewards of Low-wage Home Care Labour." *Sociology of Health and Illness* 27: 831–854.

———. 2011. *The Caring Self: The Work Experiences of Home Care Aides.* Ithaca, NY: Cornell University Press.

Tanner, Christine, Patricia Benner, Catherine Chesla, and Deborah Gordon. 1996. "The Phenomenology of Knowing the Patient." In Suzanne Gordon, Patricia Benner, and Nel Noddings (eds), *Caregiving: Readings in Knowledge, Practice, Ethics, and Politics.* Philadelphia, PA: University of Pennsylvania Press: 201–219.

Terborg-Penn, Rosalyn. 2013. "Survival Strategies among African-American Women Workers: A Continuing Process." In Ruth Milkman (ed.), *Women, Work and Protest: A Century of U.S. Women's Labor History.* New York: Routledge: 139–155.

Tolhurst, Edward, and Bernhard Weicht. 2017. "Preserving Personhood: The Strategies of Men Negotiating the Experience of Dementia." *Journal of Aging Studies* 40: 29–35.

Tolich, Martin. 1993. "Alienating and Liberating Emotions at Work: Supermarket Clerks' Performance of Customer Service." *Journal of Contemporary Ethnography* 22: 361–381.

Tronto, Joan. 2013. *Caring Democracy: Markets, Equality, and Justice.* New York: New York University of Press.

———. 1994. *Moral Boundaries: A Political Argument for an Ethic of Care.* New York: Routledge.

Vittoria, Anne K., and Mary K. Zimmerman. 2005. "The Meaning of Gender, Refuge and Resistance." Unpublished manuscript.

Vladeck, Bruce. 1980. *Unloving Care: The Nursing Home Tragedy.* New York: Basic Books.

Waerness, Kari. 1996. "The Rationality of Caring." In Suzanne Gordon, Patricia Benner and Nel Noddings (eds), *Caregiving: Readings in Knowledge, Practice, Ethics, and Politics.* Philadelphia, PA: University of Pennsylvania Press: 231–253.

West, Candace, and Don Zimmerman. 1987. "Doing Gender." *Gender and Society* 1: 125–151.
Wharton, Amy S. 1993. "The Affective Consequences of Service Work: Managing Emotions on the Job." *Work and Occupations* 20: 205–232.
Yeatts, Dale E., and Cynthia Cready. 2007. "Consequences of Empowered CNA Teams in Nursing Home Settings: A Longitudinal Assessment." *Gerontologist* 47: 323–339.
Zerubavel, Eviatar. 1979. *Patterns of Time in Hospital Life: A Sociological Perspective.* Chicago, IL: University of Chicago Press.
Zola, Irving. 1991. "Bringing Our Bodies and Ourselves Back in: Reflections on a Past, Present, and Future Medical Sociology." *Journal of Health and Social Behavior* 3: 14.
———. 1992. "The Naming Question: Reflections on the Language of Disability." In *Report of the American Association for the Advancement of Science Workshop on the Demography of Scientists and Engineers with Disabilities.* Washington, DC: American Association for the Advancement of Science: 258.

INDEX

For Product Safety Concerns and Information please contact our EU
representative GPSR@taylorandfrancis.com
Taylor & Francis Verlag GmbH, Kaufingerstraße 24, 80331 München, Germany

www.ingramcontent.com/pod-product-compliance
Ingram Content Group UK Ltd.
Pitfield, Milton Keynes, MK11 3LW, UK
UKHW022025061126
477531UK00002B/33
* 9 7 8 0 3 6 7 3 7 0 8 0 0 *